I0414487

CUTTING HEALTH CARE

CUTTING HEALTH CARE

◆

THE PROS AND CONS

Roberto C. Alvarez-Galloso, CPUR

iUniverse, Inc.

New York Lincoln Shanghai

CUTTING HEALTH CARE
THE PROS AND CONS

Copyright © 2006 by Roberto C. Alvarez-Galloso,CPUR

All rights reserved. No part of this book may be used or reproduced by any means, graphic, electronic, or mechanical, including photocopying, recording, taping or by any information storage retrieval system without the written permission of the publisher except in the case of brief quotations embodied in critical articles and reviews.

iUniverse books may be ordered through booksellers or by contacting:

iUniverse
2021 Pine Lake Road, Suite 100
Lincoln, NE 68512
www.iuniverse.com
1-800-Authors (1-800-288-4677)

ISBN-13: 978-0-595-39445-6 (pbk)
ISBN-13: 978-0-595-67707-8 (cloth)
ISBN-13: 978-0-595-83841-7 (ebk)
ISBN-10: 0-595-39445-0 (pbk)
ISBN-10: 0-595-67707-X (cloth)
ISBN-10: 0-595-83841-3 (ebk)

Printed in the United States of America

Contents

ACKNOWLEDGEMENT

I would like to thank God, My Wife Marlene, My Daughter Veronica and other Family Members for their Moral Support and Guidance in the Creation of this book.

Roberto C. Alvarez-Galloso, CPUR
Miami Florida
28-March-2006

PREFACE

The views expressed in this book are NOT of the Author, The Publishing Companies, and/or their subsidiaries.

The purpose is to discuss rationing and other alternatives in an era of constant change in the Health Care Industry.

This has been an ongoing issue for the last decades, and affects [or has affected] Health Care Professionals, Patients [Customers], Insurance Companies, and Government at all levels. Rationing [or Cutting Health Care] is a subject of Economic, Ethical, Financial, and Health Concerns.

If there is any doubt with regards to the views expressed in this book, the reader should either check the articles listed in the reference section or the laws/statutes governing his/her area of residence.

1

RATIONING: AN INTRODUCTION

Rationing can be defined as a way of limiting products in short supply in order to assure equal distribution.

World History has examples of rationing. Examples have included the USA during World War II and Cuba since 1961. Recent examples in Medicine have included Oregon, and the Czech Republic.

Recently, Great Britain [with its National Health System] has considered rationing.

According to the BBC News Article: "Rationing: 'Only Option' for NHS" [dated February 7, 2001]", the representatives of the British Medical Association, Royal College of Nursing, Patients, Private Health Care Providers, and the Pharmaceutical Industry concluded: "Increased Rationing is the only way to go forward".

BBC Look North of East Yorkshire/Lincolnshire [UK Local TV News Program] [on January 14, 2005] had a segment on how "Doctor Visits have been replaced by Paramedics".

Another general example of Cutting Health Care occurred in Turkmenistan. According to Monica Whitlock [BBC Journalist based in Central Asia], "The President of Turkmenistan ordered the closure of all hospitals in the country with the exception of Ashgabat [the capital]". Furthermore, Ms. Whitlock reported that "it was part of a health care reform in which 15,000 medical workers were replaced with army conscripts".

The Ministry of Public Health and Industry of Turkmenistan states the following: "Our Basic Activity is to Organize Preventive, Medical, Rehabilitation, Medicinal, and other kinds of Medical Aid to the Population".

Returning to the USA: In the 1990's, The US Federal Government intended to start on the task of Reforming Health Care. In 1993, Bill Clinton, [in his first acts as US President] proposed a National Health Insurance Program. The proposal was opposed by those who harped on the failure of government health insurance in other countries. The proposal was rejected by the US Congress landing Mr. Clinton one of the first defeats in his administration.

Regardless, laws such as the Consumer Bill of Rights and Responsibility and HIPAA [Health Insurance Portability and Accountability Act] were approved.

Health Care Reform was not limited to the Clinton Administration. George W. Bush [after becoming US President in 2001], decided on a Health Care Reform which would create a Paper Less Health Care System, Limit Tort Damages, Shifts Burden of Liability away from the Health Care Professionals, and a tendency towards Out Patient Clinics.

The States that form part of the USA did not wait for the [USA] Federal Government and decided to find solutions to their health care problems. Florida, [in response to high health care costs and Medicaid Expenditures] embarked on Health Care Reform during the Lawton Chiles Administration in the 1990's. Up to the present, Florida is still reforming Health Care with the possibility of making changes in its Medicaid Programs. There has been opposition from the Small Pharmacies because of fears of being "put out of business". The Underwriter has been witness to many Small Pharmacies [in Florida] installing signs [in their premises] which state: "Governor Bush, please do not privatize Medicaid". New York State approved a Health Care Reform Package in 1996 and 2000 called the New York State Health and Reform Act.

The Washington State Senate [in 2005], passed a mental health reform bill. Vermont and Ohio have also jumped on the Health Care Reform Train. According to the Heritage Foundation, "if Congress wants to reform the Health Care System, then it should reform the Health Insurance Markets".

Michigan approved a Pharmacy Reform Package. Arizona [which adopted Medicaid in 1982] and Colorado [as well as Massachusetts, & Utah] are also pursuing Health Care Reform. Indiana also adopted a prescription program. New Mexico attempted Health Care Reform yet the proposals [at the present time] have not succeeded.

It is important to place Health Care Rationing in the Discussion Table because of many factors, which include the following:

1. The Aging of The Baby Boom Generation [those who were born between 1946 to 1964].

2. The Expansion of The Human Life Span because of Recent Medical Technologies [and discoveries].

2

OREGON

The Health Plan that has received publicity in the USA [and the world] has been the Oregon Health Plan.

The Oregon Health Plan [OHP] was introduced in 1994 during the Gubernatorial Period of Ms. Barbara Roberts [Democrat] 1991-1995. The OHP is part of the Oregon Department of Human Services and is administered by the Office of Medical Assistance Program [OMAP].

The OHP offers one benefit package for all members regardless of age, and income. It offers Medicaid Benefits as well.

There are two benefit packages [which were approved by the Oregon Legislature in 2001 with the purpose of cost containment and increase availability of OHP to more Oregonians. These Two Benefit Packages are OHP Standard and OHP Plus.

OHP Standard is limited and is offered to certain adults whose qualifications are based primarily on income. In this package, premiums are paid. Since June 19, 2004, Oregonians who were covered by OHP Standard do not have to make co-payments.

OHP Standard does NOT cover the following services [at the time of writing this book]:

1. Non Emergency Transportation

2. Routine Vision Services

3. Hearing Aid Services

4. Dental Services

5. Medical Supplies and Equipment

6. Outpatient Mental Health and Substance Service

OHP Plus is a full benefit package for children, pregnant women, and disabled individuals. This package is offered at little or no cost. It does not require premiums. It does require a small co-payment for medication and outpatient services.

It must be remembered that these packages [OHP Standard and OHP Plus] are based on a prioritized list of Health Services. This list is created by the Health Services Commission and adopted by the Oregon State Legislature. This list is also subject to changes.

Although pregnant patients are covered under OHP and are not required to pay premiums, they must stay within their Medical Plan Service Area during the last 30 days of their pregnancy. Should the pregnant patient leave her Service Area, her plan will ONLY be responsible for Emergency Care OUTSIDE her area.

The Newborn Infant has Medical Coverage until he/she turns one year old, even if the mother is ineligible for OHP.

Members of OHP are able to have their family classified together as one case, in spite of family members receiving individual packages.

OHP Members can seek services from a Federally Qualified Health Clinic [FQHC] or Rural Health Clinic [RHC] if such clinics are part of the OHP Provider Panel. OHP Members are required to make a co-payment when using the FQHC and/or RHC.

Medicaid Providers in Oregon have two benefits with Managed Care:

1. Higher Reimbursement

2. Access to Highly Developed Systems.

Higher Reimbursement means that a managed care plan will pay more for services rendered for Medicaid Patients than on a Fee for Service. Patients who are not enrolled must pay the fee for service.

Access to Highly Developed Systems: Managed Care Plans that have a contract with the OHP [Oregon Health Plan] have in place a process of Continuous Quality Improvement which helps the provider address issues facing their patients and practices.

The State of Oregon Department of Human Services [taking into account Privacy Issues] has a right to use and disclose information from Enrolled Patients for:

1. Treatment

2. Payment

3. Health Care Operations

4. Appointments

5. Health Information

6. Public Health Activities

7. Inspection and/or Investigation of Health Care Providers

8. Law Enforcement

9. Investigation and Reports concerning abuse

10. Government Programs

11. Avoidance of Threat to Safety and Health of an Individual and/or the General Public

12. Research

13. Family, Friends, Significant Others [even though the person implicated can voice his/her objections]

The Patient has the right to the following:

1. See and receive his/her copy of Medical Records

2. Request a Correction and/or Update of His/Her Record

3. Receive a List of Disclosures

4. Request Limits on Disclosures and or Use of Personal Health Information [PHI]

5. Revoke Permission [Must be Done in Writing]

6. Choose Communication Methods

7. File A Complaint

8. Receive a Hard Copy of Information from the DHS

In recent developments, that in included the following:

The 2003 State Legislature mandated that the IPGB [Insurance Pool Governing Board] develop two certified plans with the intention of serving businesses that are uninsured and employ between 2 to 50 eligible employees. These two programs are: The Alternative Group Plan and The Children's Group Plan. This has also been reported by KMTR News [Oregon] in their webpage [in collaboration with Associated Press].

The Alternative Group Plan covers essential services and provides a low cost alternative to basic and catastrophic health plans existing in the commercial market. Employees and their Adult Dependents [Not Children] are covered.

The Children's Group Plan covers children up to 23 years of age. It may be purchased alone [covering only children of employees] or with the Alternative Group Plan.

The IPGB [Insurance Pool Governing Board] stated that employers may obtain premium quotes [from both plans] and start enrollment on March 1, 2005.

On October 1, 2004, OMAP [Office of Medical Assistance Program] inaugurated a One Year Pilot Program called "First Pass". The Purpose of First Pass is to process Medicaid Claims in a Timely and Accurate Fashion.

Theoretically, First Pass works like this:

1. The Provider renders health care to the patient

2. Practitioner's Office will then bill OMAP

3. OMAP will process the bill and send the payment

In practice [and taking into account that the above mentioned does not happen easily], OMAP will analyze the processes that influence provider claims [which will include time factors].

The Guiding Principles in First Pass [according to OHP First Pass Initiative] are the following:

1. Strategies, Activities, and Materials developed previous State & Private Agencies will be incorporated to the greatest extent possible.

2. Cost Effective and Affordable Solutions while Medicaid Program Provider Stakeholders receive maximum value

3. DHS Representatives will serves as facilitators within the regulatory environment

4. First Pass [& Practices by First Pass] will be independent of specific data systems

5. Complementation of DHS Program Integrity Efforts

First Pass will also support HIPAA Outreach Efforts in Electronic Billing.

First Pass will support MMIS [Medicaid Management Information System] in coordination of resources in order to foster the creation of a business improvement plan.

It should be added that the 2003-2005 Legislative Budget will provide 25 million dollars in funds for a labor contract for home care workers for the first time in Oregon's History.

There was also a partial restoration of funds for Mental Health and Addiction even though the proposed bill to increase the tax on beer was not approved by the Oregon House.

For those who are curious about the tax on Beer. One Representative [Rep. Jackie Drigfelder: D-Portland] and One Senator [Sen. Bill Morissette: D-Springfield] co sponsored a proposed bill which would increase the tax on beer [A "Cost Recovery Fee" according to them]. The logic behind this proposed bill was to raise 150 Million Dollars to fund Substance Abuse Programs. This proposal died immediately because the House Republicans [with Speaker Karen Minnis] declared that they have "No Intention of Bending the No New Tax Pledge".

Eligibility for CHIP [Children's Health Insurance Plan] was also broadened although Federal Approval for this was pending at the time this book was being written.

There are other components of the OHP [Oregon Health Plan] worth mentioning, the Oregon Medical Insurance Pool and the Family Health Insurance Assistance Program.

The Oregon Medical Insurance Pool [OMIP] was approved by the State Legislature during the period of Neil E. Goldschmidt [Democrat] as Governor [1987-1991]. The first policy was issued in July 1990. Since then, 35,000 Oregonians [who in other circumstances would not have health insurance coverage] have been insured by this program.

At the time of this writing [and subject to change], the administering insurer for OMIP is the Regence Blue Cross Blue Shield of Oregon [which handles for OMIP "eligibility, enrollment, member services, and claim processes". A Citizen's Board of Director guides OMIP Policies.

Premiums paid by enrollees are 60% of Medical and Medicine Claims Cost. Commercial Insurance Companies that do business in Oregon pay a 40% via a special fee.

It must be remembered that Individuals who are enrolled [regardless of self or family] must have the financial means to pay. OMIP does NOT subsidize or reduce premiums.

Family Health Insurance Assistance Program [FHIAP] is a program which assists Oregonian Families in their effort to obtain the benefits and protection of a health insurance plan.

FHIAP is administered by the Insurance Pool Governing Board [IGPB].

FHIAP subsidizes the purchase of Health Insurance [for qualified yet uninsured Oregonians] by paying a large part of their health insurance [by 50 to 95%]. These amounts are based on family size and income.

The requirements for FHIAP are the following:

1.   No Insurance for the previous 6 months [exception is OHP]

2.   Person is not eligible for Medicare

3.   Investments and Savings are less than $10,000

4.   Resident of Oregon who is either a US Citizen or "Qualified Non Citizen".

There exist two forms of FHIAP:

1.   Employee Sponsored Insurance

2.   Individual Insurance Plan

Employer Sponsored Insurance works via this process: If the employee increases his/her insurance at work, the employer will remove money from the paycheck. The employee has the responsibility of mailing copies of his/her pay stubs that show the amount of money withheld by the employer. FHIAP mails a reimbursement check to the employee as part of the cost.

Individual Insurance Plan: A patient on an Individual Plan can select his/her insurance company from FHIAP Lists. Once enrolled, FHIAP will bill the patient for his/her share of the premiums, and send the check [with the FHIAP subsidy] to the Insurance Company.

At the present time, [although this is subject to change] Insurance Plans approved by FHIAP are the following:

1. Health Net

2. Kaiser Permanente

3. Life Wise Health Plan of Oregon

4. ODS Health Plan of Oregon

5. OMIP [Oregon Medical Insurance Pool]

6. Pacific Source

7. Regence Blue Cross/Blue Shield of Oregon

It must be remembered that this subsidy lasts for 12 months and there are additional expenses [which includes co-payment when the patient and/or his/her family member receives medical care].

In an article by Associated Press Writer, Charles E. Beggs [March 10, 2005 and which appears in www.kgw.com], The Oregon Health Policy Committee [in a 3-2 vote] approved the Mental Health Parity Measure and sent it to the State Senate.

This measure requires health insurers to provide the same type of coverage to mental health diseases as they would to medical diseases.

Senate President Peter Courtney [Democrat-Salem] said that his priority in the legislature was "parity between mental health and physical health".

Dr. Connie Powell [Psychiatrist in Portland and Former President of the Oregon Medical Association] stated: "Mental Health Patients do not know about Insurance Restrictions on Mental Health Treatment until after help is sought."

In opposition to this measure were Senator Jeff Kruse [Republican-Roseburg] and the Associated Oregon Industry whose opposition is based on the possibility of an increase in Health Insurance Costs.

Even before the approval of this measure, the Public Employees Benefit Board was offering [since 2003] a plan in which Mental Health was paired with Physical Health in coverage. According to Kathy Loertz [spokesperson]: "Costs [with this plan] increased by less than one-half of 1%".

Other states have been looking at the Oregon Health Plan. Minnesota has talked about adopting a similar plan. [This will be discussed in a future chapter].

The Citizen's Council on Health Care [located in Minnesota] voiced their concerns which included:

1. Lack of Information for an "Informed Vote"

2. Displacement of Patient Choices and Medical Expertise by State Authorities

3. "Playing God"

4. Lack of Guarantee of Access for the Most Vulnerable

5. Laws that would "approve pain and suffering"

6. State Imposed Value Judgments

7. Overriding of Individual Ethics by State Ethics

8. Doubts of Lower Costs

9. Implementation of Decisions by Bureaucrats in the Private Sector

There was a song recorded in the 1960's or 1970's by the Rock Group: Blood, Sweat, and Tears titled: "Spinning Wheels". The verse of this song states the following: "What goes Up, Must Come Down". The same can be applied to Health Plans.

Enrollment in the OHP Standard Package was once as high as 100,000. Unfortunately, enrollment has decreased due to the following factors:

1. Changes in the Premium Requirements which went into effect on February 1, 2003.

2. Patient declining to re-enroll in OHP when their period of eligibility ends.

3. People not wanting to apply in the first place secondary to the publicity surrounding the reduction of benefits.

Premium Requirement Changes were made in an effort to make OHP operate in a way that would parallel Commercial Plans. The Payments on a Monthly Basis was required as of February 1, 2003. During the first months of the new requirements, 35,000 people were disqualified from OHP.

Gary Weeks, [Director of the Oregon Department of Human Services] sent a memorandum on the Internet [May 28, 2004]. This memorandum can be seen on the following website at: egov.oregon.gov/DHS/NEWS/MESSAGE/news/2004_05_28.shtml.

In this memorandum, the number of subscribers to OHP Standard was to be "reduced to about 20,000 by June 30, 2005".

As of July 1, 2004, the OHP Standard Plan was closed to new enrollees and those who lose their eligibility secondary to non payment of premiums and for not re applying in a timely fashion.

There were also comments [in the memorandum] about "adjustments of staffing levels to reflect these changes".

At the present time, PHP Plus Package has not been affected.

More trouble was still to come for OHP. In an article by the Associated Press Writer Niki Sullivan [which appeared in the KATU 2 News Webpage] [KATU 2 News is a local news station in Oregon] titled: "More Uninsured in Oregon as Health Plan Withers", a survey was conducted by the Oregon Progress Board [in collaboration with 16 other state agencies]. The results of this survey revealed an increasing number of Oregonians without Health Insurance [from 14% in 2002 to 17% in January 2005]. This increase in the uninsured was attributed to increase in unemployment and health care costs as well as reductions in the Oregon Health Plan [OHP].

Another survey conducted by the Oregon Medical Association in 2003 revealed that of the 4746 doctors practicing in Oregon, less than one half are accepting new patients from the Oregon Health Plan.

Mr. Alan Gustafson wrote an article in the Statesman Journal [One of Oregon's Newspapers] titled "Oregon Health Plan in Critical Condition". He wrote about how OHP had some controversy with the Medicaid Program because of certain changes on OHP that has not conformed with Medicaid. These certain modifications included "a tax on hospitals, a decrease in list of certain illnesses that could be covered". Until the Federal Government approves cuts made by the State Legislature, the OHP remain in limbo. Certain lawmakers are planning an initiative measure on the November 2006 ballot which would require the legislature [in Oregon] to "come up with a plan to extend affordable health care for more Oregonians".

The underwriter has attempted to give information that is objective and up to date about the Oregon Health Plan. If the reader wants to obtain more information before making a decision [or an opinion] about the Oregon Health Plan, please visit the following websites or write to the following institutions:

Oregon Department of Human Services/Health Services
Office of Medical Assistance Program
500 Summer Street NE E 37
Salem Oregon 97301-1079

www.dhs.state.or.us/healthplan

Citizens' Council on Health Care
1954 University Avenue West Suite 8
St Paul Minnesota 55104
E Mail: info@cchonline.org
Web Page: www.cchc-mn.org

KATU 2 News Department
2153 NE Sandy Blvd
Portland Oregon 97232
Web Page: www.katu.com

KMTR News Source 16
3825 International Court
Springfield Oregon 97477
Web Page: www.kmtr.com

KGW 8 News Channel 8
1501 SW Jefferson St.
Portland Oregon 97201
Web Page: www.kgw.com

3

MINNESOTA

As previously stated, the Oregon Health Plan has been under the microscope since its inception in 1994. Minnesota is one of the states that has taken and interest in the Oregon Health Plan.

In May 15, 2003; the Citizen's Council on Health Care [CCHC] [based in St. Paul Minnesota] issued a press release ["Minnesota Business Partnership Testifies in Support of State Imposed Health Care Rationing" stating the following: "A Public Policy Group representing 100 CEO's testified in support of Health Care Rationing". The Executive Director of the Minnesota Business Partnership Duane Benson stated: "This is consistent with what we think should be done". [Mr. Benson said this before announcing in June 2003 his resignation as Executive Director effective on October 2003. He was replaced in that position by Mr. Charlie Weaver.]

Representative Jim Abeler [Republican from Anoha Minnesota]
Responded with vehemence: "We risk greatly the welfare of the people who need your business".

Senator Berglin [Democrat from Minneapolis] stated that "It's the treatment that would not be covered."

Ms. Twila Brase [CCHC President] stated that "The business community should look to the citizens being responsible for the purchase of health care instead of seeking solutions from the state" and "It is bad business if the government had to weigh the value of the individual life and the value of individual health and treatment for those lives".

During autumn of 2003, Governor Tim Pawlenty [Republican] said: "Minnesotans deserve affordable prescription online." He instructed the State Department of Human Services Administration [along with other agencies] to look for alternatives [that are cost effective] with regards to expenses in prescription medication.

The first step was the creation of a Website [Minnesota Rx Connect Online] under the webpage: www.state.mn.us. This was to include Cost Effective Strategies and Importation of Prescription Medication from Canada.

Governor Pawlenty went on to sign "Minnesota's Best Practice Law, Chapter 288, Statute 62J.43" on May 29, 2004. The purpose of this law [which can be seen in the website: www.revisor.leg.state.mn.us/forms/getstachap.shtml] is:

1. Impose Quality of Medical Care

2. Reduce Health Care Costs

3. Encourage adoption of best practice guidelines by Physicians, Health Care Providers, and Health Plans

4. Encourage Participation in Best Practice Measurement Activity by same.

Other areas in the Minnesota Best Practices Law deals with the Responsibilities of the State Health Commissioner which are the following:

1. Identification and Promotion of Best Practices which are Physician Designed and Community Based

2. Dissemination of Information to Physicians and Other Health Care Providers on Adherence to the Best Practices in Care

3. Education of Consumers and Purchasers on effective use of information provided in the selection of providers and making wise purchasing decisions

4. Making Information about Best Practices, Quality Care Management available to "customers and participants" through the Minnesota Department of Health Website

5. Convene an Advisory Committee on Making the Department of Health Website easily accessible and user friendly.

6. Collaboration with A Non Profit Minnesota Quality Improvement Organization with specializes in Quality of Care and Best Practices in Management in order to provide criteria and assist in Data Collection

7. Development of Criteria which would include Asthma, Diabetes, and two preventive health measures such as Hypertension, and Coronary Artery Disease [which would be included for one year].

Further details about the Minnesota Best Practices Law, Chapter 288, and Statute: 621.43 were the following:

"The Commissioners of Human Services and Employee Relations may use this data for decision making processes about entering contracts with Health Care Plans.

The Commission of Health, Human Services, and Employee Relations were to submit a report to the Minnesota State Legislature before January 15, 2005 with regards to the status of "Best Practices and Quality Type Initiatives". They are also required to "present recommendations with regards to changes in statutes that would make the initiatives more effective."

"This section will not apply if the best practice guidelines authorize or recommend denial of treatment, food, or fluids necessary to sustain life on basis of age, length of life, disabilities [past, present, or predicted], degree of medical dependency, or quality of life]"

"This section expires on June 30, 2006".

On January 1, 2005, the Minnesota Department of Health submitted their report to the Minnesota Legislature. The following are outlines from the report. The full report can be seen in their webpage: http://www.health.state.mn.us/divs/fpc/HClegrpt05.pdf

However, the underwriter will give an overview of the recommendations which fall under these categories:

1. Recommendations that will require no change in Regulation

2. Recommendations for Changes in Federal Regulations [Medicare]

3. State Licensing Recommendations

4. Miscellaneous

Recommendations that will require no change in Regulations were classified under the following:

1. "Home Health Aide In-service Hours: 12 Hours Annually"

2. "Development of a Communication Plan to Inform Agencies about Medicare Conditions of Participation and Interpretive Guidelines"

3. "Improvement of Education Outreach Efforts [by the Minnesota Department of Health] using periodic reminders of resources that are available and issuing a summary of deficiencies"

4. Evaluation of the Feasibility of developing a Pre-Licensing Tutorial and Examination for Class A Home Care Providers before January 2006

5. "Education of Home Care License Applicants about the Nurse Practice Act and Legal Responsibilities of Nurses"

Recommendations for Changes to Federal Regulations [Medicare] were:

1. Collection of Outcome and Assessment Information Set [OASIS] ONLY on Medicare Clients.

2. Removal of a Lock Date with a requirement on the part of agencies to submit an OASIS Report within 30 days after completion date.

3. Changing the 5 Day Calendar Day Window to a 10 Day Calendar Window for Recertification of Medicare Clients. This would coincide with a comprehensive assessment of no later than every 60 days.

4. Changing the requirement "that a home health agency must complete a performance review of each home health aide every 12 months to annually"

5. Recognition of all Authorized Providers under state law who order medication and treatment

6. Supervision of Home Health Aide on a monthly basis.

7. Revision of Standards to allow Skilled Rehabilitation Professionals to make an Initial Evaluation Visit as well as a Comprehensive Assessment [this would include Nursing].

8. Sharing with Medicare Officials that are responsible for the Administration of Home Health Program, the State of Minnesota's Success with Tele Health Care and The Promotion of Medicare Reimbursement of such care.

9. A Brochure which would cover information for Consumers about Covered and Non Covered Medicare Services

Recommendations for State Licensing:

1. Revision of Home Care Rules in order to address the needs of consumers, create a "better overall alignment and to simplify"

2. Consideration of Electronic Signatures and Adoption of Provider's Rubber Stamps Signatures.

3. Supervision of Home Health Care Aides on a Monthly Basis

4. Promotion of a Coordination of Services which will use Hospice Regulations as a Model ["which will expand to affected licensees"]

5. Review and Consideration of Terminology in State Licensures across settings

6. Definition of Essential Services in State Licensures

7. Updating Requirements on TB Screening in order to comply with the most recent CDC Guidelines [with the elimination of repeat Chest X Rays]

Last but not least among the recommendations: Miscellaneous:

1. Fund a Study of Criminal Background Requirements.

2. Evaluation of State Licensing Fees for Home Care.

3. Survey of Class A Only Agencies on a Regular Basis.

4. Review the Need for Class B, C, E, the Board, and Lodging with Special Services Registration.

5. Study the Need to License Personal Care Provider Organizations [PCPO].

6. Explore the Possibility of Developing a Master Registry.

In August of 2002, the Minnesota Department of Health proposed regulations with the intent of beginning a state wide collection of patient data.

This proposed regulation was removed [on March 3, 2003] because of opposition from certain legislators. Yet the attempt to remove this proposal was blocked by Health Officials of Governor Pawlenty [Republican] and HHS Finance Chair Rep. Fran Bradley [Republican-Rochester].

Governor Pawlenty created the Health Cabinet called Maximum Strength Health Care in late 2003. Its purpose was to report Health Care Issues and Make Recommendations. There are six commissioners of State Departments working together:

1. Department of Employee Relations [Chair]

2. Department of Health

3. Department of Labor and Industry

4. Department of Commerce

5. Department of Human Services

6. Department of Finances

Gov. Pawlenty has asked his Health Cabinet to "examine the buying power of the State and Private Sector with the intention of making substantive changes to Minnesota's Health Care Purchasing System and Costs. Ways will be examined in how the State of Minnesota could use its role as a Health Care Provider and Regulator to reduce Health Care Costs and Improve Quality of Care".

The Health Cabinet was organized into 4 Main Work Groups [which will lead by one or more than one Health Cabinet Member]. Each Work Group was to utilize State Staff, Consult outside Experts, and make recommendations to the Governor.

This may lead to legislative proposals when the Minnesota Legislature holds it session in 2005.

The opportunities to provide input would be by the following:

1. Public Meetings and Forums

2. Meeting with Groups and Experts

3. Formation of the Health Cabinet Website

    I. Public Meetings and Forums:

    > 1. A number of forums and meetings are being planned with the intention of maintaining the people of Minnesota informed of the Health Cabinet's Work.

    > 2. It will be an opportunity to provide feedback and proposals of ideas.

    II. Meeting with Groups and Experts:

    > 1. The Health Cabinet and Work Group associated with it will meet with a variety of groups representing interests related to health care business and citizens. [This will include Outside Experts].

    III. Health Cabinet Website:

    > 1. Creation of the website with the title: www. MaximumStrengthHealthCare.com with the intention of providing information, updates, and a calendar of meetings.

    > 2. The website will also offer opportunities for the people of Minnesota to comment and propose ideas.

Many departments exist within the Minnesota Health Care System:

1. Minnesota Care

2. General Assistance Medical Care [GMAC]

3. Minnesota Senior Health Options [MSHO]

4. Prescription Drugs and Medicare Related Programs

We will now enter into a lengthy discussion of each department.

Under Minnesota Care, the following services for enrollees are covered:

1. Doctor and Health Clinic Visits for Preventive/Non Preventive Care.

2. Family Planning

3. Immunizations

4. Laboratories

5. X Ray Services

6. Outpatient Surgery

7. Chiropractic Care

There are Co-Payments [which are subject to change] for the following services:

1. Eye Glasses, Mental Health Services, Emergency Room Visits for some Adults without Children

2. Prescription for some adults without children [although Co-Payments may be lower for non pregnant adults].

What will not be paid are the following services:

1. Cosmetic Surgery

2. Autopsy [Necropsy]

3. Missed Appointments

4. Vocational Educational Services

5. Artificial In Vitro Insemination [including Fertility Drugs]

There is also a calendar year limit [subject to change as well] for services that are covered.

Additional Services during a Hospitalization that can be covered are:

1. Alcohol and Chemical Dependence Treatment

2. Medical Equipment and Supplies

3. Rehabilitative Therapy

4. Eye Glasses

5. Dental Service

Dental Services may be covered with a limit of $500.00 per year. This will exclude Emergency Services, Dentures, and Extractions before dentures. There will be a Co Payment for Restorative Dental Services [Fillings or False Teeth].

There are asset limits for families of one, two, or more [this is also subject to change]. There is no asset limits for pregnant women or children under 21.

The most commonly common assets are:

1. Cash

2. Savings Accounts

3. Checking Accounts

4. Certificate of Deposits

5. Stocks

6. Bonds

7. Motor Vehicles used for Non Employment Purposes

8. Recreational Vehicles

9. Land and/or Horses not utilized

10. Amount of Capital of a trade or business exceeding $200,000 [in 2004]

Assets that would not be counted:

1. The home a person lives in

2. Household or Personal Goods

3. Motor Vehicles used for Employment Purposes

4. Individually Owned Pension and Retirement Funds

Eligibility in Minnesota Care depends on whether the person meets the following qualifications:

1. Social Security Number

2. Residency in Minnesota [person must have lived in Minnesota for six months, if the person is an adult without children or whose children are over 21 years of age]

3. Absence of other Health Insurance [which would include Medicare] for at least four months. [The exception to this rule has been enrollees of Medical Assistance whose Health Insurance has been paid by Medical Assistance].

Another qualification that can be included is if the person is unable to obtain Health Insurance through an employer who would pay at least the monthly cost.

The present income levels in Minnesota Care are effective through June 30, 2005. These limits increase every July 1st.

For Pregnant Women and Children under 21: [Minnesota Care]

Family Size including Unborn	Income Limit [Monthly Gross]
1	$2134
2	$2863
3	$3592
4	$4321
5	$5050
Additional	Add $729

Adults over 21, NO Children

Family Size	Income Limit [Monthly Gross]
1	$1358
2	$1822

Parents, Legal Guardians, Foster Parents, and Relative Caretakers of Children under 21 have the same income limits. An exception to this is a family size of 4 or more [in which their income level is $4166 and they are illegible if Gross Annual Income exceeds $50,000]

The next topic to be discussed will be General Assistance Medical Care [GMAC]. GMAC has two levels of covered services:

1.   Comprehensive Benefits

2.   Hospital Only

Comprehensive Benefits provide coverage for:

1.   Preventive Care [History and Physical Examination included]

2.   Immunization

3.   Family Planning

4.   Laboratory Services

5.   Radiology Services

6.   Emergency Room [during Emergency Care]

7.   Inpatient Hospitalization

8.   Outpatient Surgery

9.   Medical Equipment

10.   Medical Samples

11.   Rehabilitation

12. Mental Health Services

13. Substance Abuse Treatment

14. Prosthetics

15. Hearing Aids

16. Health Insurance Premiums that are Cost Effective

17. Prescription Medication [which would include Birth Control Pills]

Comprehensive Coverage in GMAC may be effective on the date that the county human service agency receives a signed and dated application plus a written request for coverage.

There is exists a $3.00 Co Payment for Brand Name Medications and a $1.00 Co Payment for Generic Brand. The Maximum Co Payment allowed is $20.00.

The following services under GMAC have a $3.00 Co Payment Visits:

1.   Clinic and Physician Services for Non Preventive Care

2.   Chiropractic Care

3.   Podiatry

4.   Audiology

5.   Ophthalmologic [Eye] Examinations.

The following services have a $25.00 Co Payment:

1.   Eye Glasses

2.   Emergency Room Visits for Non Emergency Care

Dental Coverage is $500 per Calendar Year. Exceptions are Emergency Dental Services and Dentures/Extractions.

Hospitalization ONLY under GMAC may begin on the day of hospitalization or on the day the application is submitted to the county human service agency. Coverage ends on the day of discharge. The person must be currently hospitalized or expect to be hospitalized within 45 days from the date the last application is submitted.

GMAC Hospitalization covers the following:

1. Inpatient Hospitalization Services [A Co Payment of $1000 applies to each admission]

2. Physician Services received during hospitalization

GMAC Hospitalization DOES NOT Cover:

1. Cosmetic Surgery

2. Autopsy [Necropsy]

3. Missed Appointments

4. Vocational Services

5. Educational Services

6. Gender Reassignment Surgery

7. Artificial or In Vitro Insemination [including Fertility Drugs]

GMAC Requirement for eligibility is the following:

1. Person cannot be eligible for Medical Assistance.

2. Person must live in Minnesota for at least 30 days and intends to stay.

3. Is a US Citizen [or a Non Citizen who is residing lawfully in the USA]

GMAC has income limits. This Income Eligibility is based on Gross Income received during a six month period. This [Income Eligibility] changes once a year in July.

The present limits are in effect until June 30, 2005.
GMAC Comprehensive Coverage Income Limits

Family Size	Limits
1	$3492
2	$4686
3	$5880
4	$7074

Additional Members $1194

GMAC Hospitalization Only Coverage Income Limits

Family Size	Limits
1	$8148
2	$10432
3	$13716
4	$16500

Additional Members are $2784 more

GMAC also has Asset Limits:

1. Comprehensive Coverage of $1000 for families of any size.

2. Hospitalization Only Coverage of $10,000 for a family of one and $20,000 for families of two or more.

In GMAC, the most commonly counted assets are:

1. Savings Accounts

2. Checking Accounts

3. Certificate of Deposits

4. Stocks

5. Bonds

6. Recreational Vehicles

7.   Land or houses that the person does NOT Live on

Non Counted Assets are:

1.   The house a person lives in

2.   Household and Personal Goods

3.   Motor Vehicles under certain conditions

4.   Capital and Operational Assets of a Trade or Business

For GMAC Hospitalization Coverage, Non Counted Assets are:

1.   Vehicles used for Employment Purposes

2.   Individually Owned Pension and Retirement Funds

In GMAC Hospitalization Only Coverage, enrollees are limited to $200,000 in capital operating assets.

Minnesota Senior Health Option Program [MSHO] is a program for the population that is 65 years of age and older [senior citizens] [who are eligible for Medicare and Medical Assistance]. Only those individuals over 65 years of age that have Medical Assistance can join.

MHSO combines health care and support services from different programs into one.

There is no additional cost to join and senior citizens have the option of joining MHSO or remaining with their Medical Assistance [MA] Program.

MHSO is administered by the Minnesota Department of Human Services in partnership with Medica Metropolitan Health Plan, and U Care [This is the current arrangement at the time of writing this chapter and may be subject to change].

MHSO is also overseen by the Center for Medicare and Medicaid Services [CMS] and has received funds and other forms of assistance from the Robert Wood Johnson Foundation.

The enrollee must choose a Health Plan. The Health Plan assigns a Care Coordinator for each enrollee to assist with the paperwork access health care and support services.

The patient [client] can leave MHSO by notifying the agency in Writing. Afterwards, the Department of Human Services will then remove the patient out of MHSO at the beginning of next month.

Medical Assistance [MA] in the Minnesota Health Care Program are for people who are 65 years and older, disabled, Children under 21, pregnant women, and parents/relative caretakers of dependent children.

Income Limits vary taking into account family size, age, blindness, other disabilities, or pregnancy.

Some enrollees have only a limited amount of assets. Asset Limits are non existent for pregnant women and children under the age of 21.

Covered Health Services in MA include the following:

1. Doctor's Visit

2. Hospitalization

3. Prescriptions

4. Dental Care

5. Eye Examination

There is no cost for those who meet the income limit, although some services may require a co payment. If the patient's income exceeds the limit, he/she may still qualify for payment of certain medical costs

Another part of the Minnesota Health Care System is the Prescription Drug Program and other programs related to Medicare.
Patients who are enrolled in Medicare [which is a Federal Program for Citizens over 65 years of age and/or with disability] are eligible.

The Income Limits may vary taking into account the size of the family and the programs. The programs are the following:

1. Qualified Medicine Beneficiary Program [QMB]

2. Service Limited Medicare Beneficiary Program [SLMB]

3. Prescription Drug Program [PDP]

4. Qualified Individual Group 1 Program [Q1-1]

5. Qualified Working Disabled Program [QWD]

The services are limited and may vary depending on program enrollment.

1. QMB, SLMB, and Q1-1 pay the premium for Medicare Part B.

2. QWD pays the Medicare A Premiums.

3. QMB cover Medicare A Premium Co-Payment and Deductible.

4. PDP covers only the prescription medication and enrollees [at the time of this writing] pay the first $35.00 in prescription costs every month.

5. There are no costs for QMB, SLMB, Q1-1, and/or QWD.

The asset limits of these above mentioned plans [in 2004] are the following: PDP, QMB, SLMB, and Q1-1

1. $10,000 for a person living alone.

2. $18,000 for a married couple and/or family.

QWD

1. $4000 for a person who lives alone.

2. $6000 for a married couple and/or family

On September 9, 2004, A News Release from the United Stated Department of Health and Human Services [HHS] announced that HHS approved a plan by Minnesota and Hawaii to save money on Prescription Medications. Under this plan, Minnesota and Hawaii would form joint purchasing pools for their Medicaid Programs. This plan would save Minnesota Tax Payers $14 Million Dollars and Hawaii $4.1 Million Dollars off Prescription Medication prices bought by these states via their programs.

With this announcement, Minnesota and Hawaii joined Michigan, Vermont, New Hampshire, Alaska, and Nevada in a Multidisciplinary Pool which allowed states to come together and negotiate lower prices on Medications purchased for their State Medicaid Program.

In the year 2005, [January 1, 2005]: Minnesota was at a crossroads with the Health Care System. Minnesota faced a budget deficit of at least $700 Million Dollars. Minnesota Legislators [along with Governor Pawlenty and House Republicans] decided to target increasing government health costs in its battle with the deficit. Governor Pawlenty declared: "Minnesota could be bankrupt in less than 15 years."

Representative Fran Bradley [Republican from Rochester] proposed a merger of Medical Assistance, Minnesota Care, and General Assistance Medical Care in order to "eliminate inefficiency". Rep. Bradley also proposed using money destined for Minnesota Care in order to cover the costs from other Government Health Programs.

Senator Linda Berglin [DFL from Minneapolis] [Head of the Senate Health and Human Services Budget Committee blames the increasing health costs on Cuts to State Programs and has proposed reversing the cuts.

It must be remembered that MA, GMAC, Minnesota Care together cover more than 666,000 Minnesotans. This is a 26% Increase since 2000. The Department of Human Services expects an increase to about 721,000 by the year 2009.

After the Federal Government ordered Minnesota to notify its citizens of who qualified for MA [Medical Assistance], some Recipients of Minnesota Care switched to MA. One of the reasons for this switch is that MA Recipients do not have to pay premiums and receive most Medical Services than Minnesota Care.

Minnesota is also projecting an increase of almost 20% in MA [with eligibility reaching 575,000 a month by 2009] and a decrease of almost 40% in Minnesota Care [to 89,000].

GMAC has a projection of an increase enrollment of about 50% [56,000] by the year 2009.

The legislature is also looking into the possibility of a higher cigarette tax with the intention of using the money [collected from such a tax] to reduce health taxes for small businesses. Another alternative could be a ban on smoking in Minnesota or a No Fault Health Insurance for those unable to afford Private Health Insurance but cannot qualify for State Programs. Governor Pawlenty and his Health Cabinet have been studying the No Fault Insurance Issue by looking at programs in Massachusetts and New York.

On January 27, 2005, an article from the Associated Press appeared in the WCCO [A Radio and Television Station in Minneapolis/St. Paul Minnesota] webpage. In this article "Six Insurance Plans to be offered for Uninsured" [which appears on the webpage: http://wcco.com/localnews/ local_story_027200229.html] HR Policy Association announced the formation of six health insurance plans [for those who are Part Time Workers, Contractors, and Early Retirees and do not qualify for Corporate Health Insurance] by a consortium of large companies [such as Ford Motor Company and Sears].

Workers were to be offered a choice of benefits from Full Insurance Policies to those that will cost $4.41 a month. United Health Group is to offer the less expensive plan while Major Medical Policies will be handled by Humana Inc. and Cigna Corp. [Two Health Insurance Companies]. Premiums will be variable.

Mark Lindsey [who is the United Health Group Spokesman] stated: "We're not doing it to be profitable. We're doing it because we realize that having 45 Million People who are uninsured is terrible for the Health Care System."

On January 26, 2005 [in an article from the WCCO Website and written by Associated Press], Minnesota Hospitals expressed fears about the impact of Governor Pawlenty's Cuts in State Health Programs.

The cuts were to remove Childless Adults and some parents from Minnesota Care. These were eligible to switch if:

1. Income Levels were below Poverty Levels.

2. Patient [Client] Income was lowered to Poverty Level by Tendering Payment of Medical Bills.

According to the Department of Human Services, these cuts will affect 26,000 people by 2007. According to the Democratic Farmer Labor Party in Minnesota [DFL], these cuts would affect 40,000 people.

A Survey conducted by the Minnesota Hospital Association [of 77 hospitals in Minnesota] revealed that Uncompensated Hospital Care increased by 28% in 2004.

For those who are curious, Uncompensated Hospital Care includes debts that cannot be collected from patients [who cannot pay] and charity care. In this case, hospitals pass the cost through higher health insurance premiums. Non Profit Hospitals pass the cost via Higher Property Taxes.

In the year 2004, when Uncompensated Care increased 38% to $31.4 Million in Hennepin County Medical Center, property was taxed for $19.4 Million.

Uncompensated Care increased to 38% at Regions Hospital in St. Paul and 31% at North Country Health Services in Bemidji, Minnesota.

James Hanko [CEO and President of North Country Health Services] stated the following in response to the Health Care Cuts: "Health Care Cuts enacted by this state [Minnesota] 2 years ago are a dominant factor in the rise of uncompensated care."

On February 26, 2005, Associated Press and WCCO TV reported about a study by the University of Minnesota [commissioned by the Minnesota Department of Health]. In this study, [in 2001] 5.4% of Minnesotans lacked private or public health insurance. This percentage increased to 6.7% by the year 2004.

This report also revealed that fewer Minnesotans received health coverage in their place of work. [This was a result of employees scaling back benefits].

Between the years 2001 to 2004, the state reduced its spending on subsidized health care programs for the working poor. At the same time, health costs were increasing at a double digit rate with each year. Minnesotans in State Programs increased from 10% in 2001 to 15% in 2004.

It is predicted by the expert in the Health Care Field that taking into account that those without insurance will most likely seek emergency care that is costly, taxpayers and health insurance companies will be most affected.

Senator Linda Berglin [DFL-Minneapolis] declared that "The situation was a death spiral."

Bruce Rueben [Executive Director of the Minnesota Hospital Association stated: "You can't keep people from being sick just because they don't have insurance."

An I-Team Coverage Report by Terri Grucca, [March 2, 2005] [based on figures which WCCO obtained from the Mayo Clinic with prices subject to change] revealed the following:
Private Room:

- Allina : $1390

- Mayo: $1070

- Methodist: 1524

For a Colonoscopy:

- Allina: $1455

- Mayo: $3300

- Methodist: $1524

For a Caesarian Section [C-Section]:

- Allina: $16,922

- Mayo: $17,750

- Methodist: $14,004

In an interview with WCCO—TV, Allina Hospital Spokespeople stated the following: "Money will not get in the ay of care. Financial Counselors will help foot the bill"

In other developments, Minnesota's Drug Program with Canada continued to expand with one program [Minnesota Senior Federation] added to Medi Save Discount Pharmacy.

February 16, 2005: [In an article by the Associated Press and appearing in the WCCO Webpage] Governor Tim Pawlenty discussed the possibility of Native American Tribes in Northern Minnesota acting as wholesale purchasers of prescription medication from Canada. This was in response to the possibility of the FDA [Food and Drug Administration] and Canada restricting cross border medication.

A spokesperson for the Native American Community stated that they conversed with Canada concerning this subject. The spokesperson also stated that the Native American Community was doing a feasibility study on importation of medications.

In response to the possibility of a restriction and/or shutdown of cheaper medication from Canada by the Canadian Government or the FDA, Senior Citizens Groups [Minnesota Senior Federation and Coalition of Wisconsin Aging Group] met in Philadelphia Pennsylvania with the intention of discussing the possibility of importing prescription medication outside of North America.

March 10, 2005: Governor Pawlenty considered the possibility of importing prescription medications from certain pharmacies in Great Britain. State Workers were sent to Great Britain to study such a possibility and make recommendations.

March 15, 2005: In an AARP [American Association of Retired People] Meeting: Governor Pawlenty announced that while looking for cheaper prescription medication beyond US Borders was not "a broad solution for the whole country", "Congress approved a bill that would prohibit Medicare from negotiating bulk agreements which would have lead to deeper discounts".

March 18, 2005: Governor Pawlenty announced [after the commission's trip to Great Britain and subsequent report] that he approved adding British Pharmacies to Minnesota's Rx Connect Program. The US Food and Drug Administration criticized this as "an ill considered expansion of a risky program". Regardless, FDA has no plans to block Minnesota at the present time.

[Before continuing, an article by the Associated Press made public a report by Larsen, Weishair, and Company [Accounting Firm based in Minneapolis Minnesota which works on behalf of half of the Nursing Homes in Minnesota]. This report stated that because of financial losses that exceed 5%, 25% of the Nursing Homes in the state are at risk of closing.]

March 29, 2005: A Bill backed by Ms. Sheila Kiscaden; Independent-Rochester and Mr. Jim Abeler; Republican-Anoha would require Minnesotans to buy basic health insurance coverage. This would start in the year 2007. [This bill was proposed by the Minnesota Medical Association]. It would have Minnesotans paying the same premium for basic medical benefits with the purpose of risk spreading statewide. This bill would require proof of health insurance to be present in tax returns and driver's license's renewal.

March 31, 2005: The Minnesota Senate votes 43 to 17 to lift a gap on health care expenses for childless adults enrolled in a government insurance health program. Senator Linda Berglin [Democratic Farmer Labor-Minneapolis] sponsored the bill with the reason that "caps treat these folks [childless adults] like second class citizens. Opponents of this measure responded that "The State of Minnesota cannot afford limitless care while coping with a budget deficit."

April 1, 2005: The Minnesota Senate also voted [on March 31, 2005] to restore certain health care funding for working adults without children. This appeared in the article by the Associated Press dated April 1, 2005 on the website of WCCO. [http://wcco.com/health/local_story_091094049.html]

April 4, 2005: Shareholders of the largest pharmaceutical companies in the USA will vote at the end of April on a resolution sponsored by the Minnesota to "quit restricting supplies to Canadian Pharmacies" that have US Citizens as customers. The Pharmaceutical Companies responded by talking about the dangers of "imported drugs".

April 12, 2005: AARP [American Association of Retired People] [in its annual pharmaceutical report] commented about an increase by 7.1% in the price of brand name prescription medication.

April 19, 2005: Minnesota House Republicans unveiled a Spending Bill which would make deepening cuts to Public Insurance Programs. [These cuts were more than what was proposed by Governor Pawlenty: Republican]. These cuts were to occur during the Budget Period of 2006 and 2007.

April 27, 2005: A study funded by the Robert Wood Johnson Foundation [using data from the USA Center for Disease Control and Prevention; 2003] revealed that Minnesota [compared with the rest of the USA], had the lowest percentage of people without health insurance. Minnesota was also first when it came to lowest uninsured rates for adults with jobs.

May 4, 2005: Shareholders of the three largest manufacturers of pharmaceutical medications reject the resolution of Minnesota with regard to importation of medications. The $8.7 Billion Health Package expanding Minnesota Care Insurance passes in the Democratic Controlled Senate by 38 votes to 29.

The Health Care Landscape in Minnesota is in constant evolution. No one book or article can hope to cover everything. Again, the reader can obtain more information by visiting the following:

Minnesota North Star
State of Minnesota Online
Web Page: http://www.state.mn.us/

Minnesota Department of Health
P.O.Box 64975
St. Paul Minnesota 55164-0975
Web Page: http://www.health.state.mn.us

Citizens' Council on Health Care
1954 University Avenue West Suite 8
St Paul Minnesota 55104
E Mail: info@cchonline.org
Web Page: www.cchc-mn.org

WCCO TV 4 News
90 South 11th Street
Minneapolis Minnesota 55403
Web Page: www.wcco.com

4

TENNESSEE

Another Health Care Program worth mentioning is Tenn Care.

Tenn Care is Tennessee's Managed Health Care Program that provides health care benefits to the following:

1. Medicaid Beneficiaries

2. Uninsured Children

3. Consumers with Medical Conditions that have rendered them uninsurable.

Tenn Care was established in 1994 as a Cost Effective Health Program. Before the establishment of Tenn Care, Costs for the Medicaid Program was increasing out of proportion.

1. 1969: Medicaid Spending consumed 3% of Tennessee's Budget

2. 1993: Medicaid Spending consumed 26% of its budget.

The increases in health care costs had a domino effect, a rise in uninsured people. The Uninsured People get sick, "receive charity care" at a hospital; the charity care became expensive for hospitals, doctors, and state [the last one reimbursing the facilities]

Tenn Care is divided into two components:

1. Physical Health

2. Mental Health and Substance Abuse

The Physical Health Component is managed by MCO's [Managed Care Organizations].

The Mental Health and Substance Abuse Component are managed by Behavioral Care Organizations.

Tenn Care is funded like most Medicaid Programs; for every dollar that is spent by the state on health care, the state receives two dollars from the Federal Government [at the time of this writing].

Tennessee bundles together the uninsurable [poor health] with uninsured [secondary to lack of access]. Tennessee would then receive Federal Money "Match" that would cover more people.

Tenn Care managed to save money for Tennessee with the following:

1.   Keeping down Medical Costs through Medicare.

2.   Emphasis on Primary and Preventive Care [which would decrease the need for emergency room visits and expensive medical care].

3.   Because of the huge number of enrollees, Tenn Care has been able to negotiate better rates for prescription medications [and other items]

4.   Tennessee has been able to receive more Federal Matching Funds to cover most of its citizens.

It should be worth mentioning that Tenn Care is NOT A FREE RIDE. Those that have the means to tender payment will do so by paying premiums based on incomes. These premiums can be compared to a private insurance plan. It is also worth remembering that some part of Tenn Care is funded partially by those who pay premiums.

Unfortunately, Tennessee has not escaped the wrath of economic malaise that has affected other states in the USA.

2004: Governor Bredesen [Democrat] outlined his strategy for Tenn Care Reform. He states that "reforms cannot be achieved without relief from constraints".

May 2004: The Tenn Care Reform Legislation is passed by the Tennessee General Assembly with almost unanimous support. The Tennessee Justice Center takes the State to Court in an "attempt to block reform effort".

September 2004: Tennessee submits a formal waiver application to the Federal Government.

Three Alternatives Plans were presented:

1. Original Preferred Path.

2. Revert To Medicaid.

3. Basic Tenn Care.

Original Preferred Path:

1. Preserves Enrollment.

2. Protects Children, Pregnant Women, and the Disabled.

Revert to Medicaid:

1. Return to Medicaid

2. Remove 430,000 People [which would also include 112,000 children] from the program.

Basic Tenn Care:

1. Stop Short of Basic Medicaid with the creation of a two tiered system that preserves coverage for 112,000 children.

Overview of the Scaled Back Program:

1. Continuation of Tenn Care via Medicaid including an expansion population for 112,000 children.

2. Implementation of Benefits for Most Adults in Medicaid Program.

3. Reduction of Enrollment in the Expansion Population with the provision of only basic services to remaining Medicaid Eligible Adults.

4. 75% of those enrolled would remain on program

5. Return to Managed Care Concept

6. Challenging Consent Decrees in Federal Courts since changes are needed for long term cost containment.

November 10, 2004: According to the News Max.com Wires, Governor Phil Bredesen announced that he will eliminate Tenn Care and revert to the traditional Medicaid Program. Governor Bredesen also announced that he would need Federal Approval and a 60 day notification period.

The Tennessee Justice Center [an organization who is leading the battle in the court for maintenance of Tenn Care] replied in a statement: "The Lawsuits will not go away. If he [Bredesen] were to do what he threatened to do, [eliminate Tenn Care] 1 Tennessean will die every 16 hours".

An Independent Study predicted that "with no changes in Tenn Care, Health Care Costs may consume 40% of the State Budget by 2005."

January 11, 2005: Governor Bredesen reduced Tenn Care Benefits to 719,000. This spared the children [who were under Tenn Care] from the reductions. Unfortunately, the cuts eliminated health care coverage for nearly half of the adults that were enrolled in Tenn Care.

The Center on Budget and Policy Priorities did a study on Tenn Care titled: "The Potential Impact of Eliminating Tenn Care and Reverting to Medicaid: A Preliminary Analysis." The authors were Leighton Ku and Vikki Wachino. This analysis can be found in the website: www.cbpp.org.

The results from this analysis were the following:

1. Elimination of Tenn Care will NOT produce a substantial amount of savings unless there are substantial cuts in health care services for those eligible for Medicaid.

2. The reversion to a Traditional Medicaid Program will cause a twice as much loss in Federal Funding. This would lead to a reduction [substantial] of employment and business activity in Tennessee.

3. Financial Problems of a severe nature for Health Care Providers in Tennessee.

January 29, 2005: US District Court Judge William J. Haynes Jr. ruled that Governor Bredesen could NOT remove 323,000 Adults from Tenn Care without consulting the Courts.

According to the State of Tennessee Tenn Care Website: "Tenn Care: Changing Tenn Care in an Adversarial Legal Environment", Tennessee was to begin a timetable in 2005 [and taking into account approval from CMS: Center for Medicare and Medicaid Services of the US Federal Government] which would:

1. Gain Relief from Consent Degrees through Legal Effort.

2. Remove Non Medicaid "Dual Eligible" and Uninsured Adults.

3. Freeze Enrollment of "Adult Expansion Enrollees" [which includes: "Adult Non Pregnant Medically Needy Spend down Population].

4. End of Pharmacy Benefits for Adults in "Expansion Populations"

5. Implement a 4 Prescription Limit for Adults in Medicaid.

6. Removal of Uninsurable Adults.

7. "Assess Broader Non Pharmacy Benefit limits for Adult Enrollees of Medicaid.

February 7, 2005: A survey by the University of Tennessee Center for Business and Economic Research revealed that in 2004; 67,772 young adults in Tennessee lacked health insurance. This was a 3% increase from 2003. Another study from the Center of Budget and Policy Priority revealed an increase of 9% in Children lacking Health Insurance among the working poor [which are families who earn 100 to 200% of the US Federal Poverty Level]. Dr. Scott Morris [founder and Executive Director of Church Health Center stated that visits to the [Church Health] Center by Uninsured Children doubled between 2003 and 2004. Dr. Morris added that "many of these children once qualified for Tenn Care."

February 10, 2005: Two Events:

1. A Federal Judge [USA] ruled in favor of Tenn Care Enrollees that were tapped for elimination from the Expanded Medicaid Program. The ruling was whether Gordon Bonneyman could remain [or not] as the Principle Attorney for the Enrollees.

2. AARP in Tennessee declared that the proposed "cuts in Tenn Care were devastating". AARP proposed to the governor as an alternative for reform; the use of generic medications [instead of brand names] and community based or in home care for elderly and disabled citizens.

February 11, 2005: Dr. Peter Chyka [Professor of Pharmacy at the University of Tennessee Health Center in Memphis, TN] stated that proposed changes in limiting prescriptions could affect health care for people with private health insurance. [It should be remembered [2005] that Tennessee was 17 to 18 prescriptions per year, Tenn Care was 30 prescriptions per year, The National Average for Prescriptions were 10 a year]. Andy Schneider [Policy Analyst with Medicaid Policy LLC based in Washington DC disagreed with Dr. Chyka. His disagreement was based on the reason that "Physicians who serve Medicaid Patients are usually different from Physicians who serve the rest of the population." Dr. Terry Shea [Director of Pharmacy Management for Blue Cross Blue Shield of Tennessee] stated that prescription limits on a monthly basis would reduce Tennessee's Dubious Image as the leading consumers of prescription medications in the USA. Ms. Wanda Moebius [Spokesperson for the Pharmaceutical Research and Manufacturers of America] stated that prescription medication reform may increase health care costs.

February 13, 2005: [Taken from an article by the Associated Press and which appeared on the website of WSMV: a Television Station in Nashville Tennessee]. Officials declared that hospitals would have to increase service rates at 17% in order to offset $660 Million in Charity Care if Tenn Care Reform Takes place. Blue Cross Blue Shield Of Tennessee Spokesperson Bill Steverson commented on how hospitals have asked BCBS to increase payments [to hospitals] by 15% as part of a Tenn Care Surcharge.

February 13, 2005 [Continued]: Craig Becker [President of the Tennessee Hospital Association] stated that hospital rates would increase which are about 5% and would be used to offset lost revenue.

February 17, 2005: The Middle Tennessee State University Poll Conducted between February 3, 2005 to February 11, 2005 gave Governor Bredesen a 62% approval rating [up from 1% in October 2004]. The same poll revealed that 53% of those polled were against Tenn Care Reform.

February 18, 2005: Tenn Care Lawyers requested a Speedy Hearing with the 6th US Circuit Court of Appeals with regards to Tenn Care Reform on the basis of the separation of power between the State Government and US Federal Government.

February 25, 2005: The Tenn Care Story took a comic turn when Tenn Care Officials told Senator Jerry Cooper [Chairman of the Senate Commerce, Labor, and Agricultural Committee] that the General Assembly will have to pay between $70,000 and $75,000 for records. This was after the General Assembly asked Tenn Care for the Records. Dave Goetz [Finance Commissioner] justified the costs by saying "Seven Weeks of Senior Staff Time, Program Work will cost between $70,000 and $75,000. The reply of Senator Cooper was: "I will recover the money with a deduction from the Tenn Care Budget. They [Tenn Care] want to play chicken, we will play chicken".

February 25, 2005 to March 7, 2005: In another saga of the Tenn Care Story. Senator John Ford reportedly received $237,000 in consulting fees from Managed Care Service Group. [Managed Care Service Group was an interest group hired by Doral Dental Services with the intention of having a contract with Tenn Care]. The Senate Ethics Committee investigated John Ford for possible breach, conflict of interest in the deal. Governor Bredesen challenged all agencies with Tenn Care Contracts to "come out clean with intent to reveal improper conduct". The Registry of Election Finance, The Office of the Attorney General, and the FBI [Federal Bureau of Investigation] also began investigations. This scandal has affected Harold Ford Jr. [a US Representative] since his career has been damaged by revelations about his Uncle's Conduct [even though he was not accused of wrongdoing]. On April 20, 2005, Tenn Care announced the cancellation of its contract with Doral Dental. The reason given was Doral's Tie with State Senator

John Ford. On May 6, 2005: Senator Ford told the Memphis Flyer [a Newspaper] that he will not run for reelection.
May 28, 2005: John Ford resigns from the Senate.

March 18, 2005: US District Judge William J. "Joe" Haynes Jr. told attorneys on both sides of the Tenn Care Reform Act Case that there will be a "sweeping review" of Governor Bredesen's Reform Package. Judge Haynes stated to the lawyers that his review will be based on 5 subjects:

1. The History of Compliance in good faith by Tennessee with consent degrees.

2. If proposed changes in Tenn Care violates US Federal Law.

3. Whether Lawyers on both sides of the Tenn Care issue bargained in good faith

4. Were the proposed changes "suitably tailored in response to changed circumstances in Tennessee?

5. Were "reasonable alternatives" adequately explored to preserve benefits for enrollees protected by Consent Decrees?

March 25, 2005: The United States Center for Medicare and Medicaid Services approved the first phase of Governor Bredesen's Tenn Care Reform, [which was the removal of 323,000 people from Tenn Care].

March 28, 2005: Gordon Bonneyman [Lawyer for those challenging the Tenn Care Reform] promised that he will prove to the courts that Governor Bredesen "mismanaged Tenn Care and he wants to shift the blame to the Courts".

March 31, 2005: Senator Ron Ramsey of Blountsville [Senate Republican Leader] commented on the need for legislative involvement in Tenn Care. He stated that "the governor had two years to reform the program and is polling to make sure that Tenn Care Reform does not hurt him in the polls." He also added: "This will become a political issue…I don't think that last year when he said that he would kick 323,000 people off that people would consider it as reform.
Dr. Bruce Steinhauer [President and CEO of the Regional Medical Center in Memphis Tennessee] stated [before Judge William J. "Joe" Haynes in the Tenn

Care Crisis] that there exists "medically needy people" who need Tenn Care. He also added that hospitals would lose without Tenn Care because people without insurance would have to be treated.

The Tennessean [a newspaper] reported about how the Bredesen Administration budgeted $48 Million less for medications than in Fiscal Year 2004. The Plan was 4 Prescriptions a month. State Officials never sought permission for the prescription limits from the US Federal Government.

April 4, 2005: Hearings in the Court of US District Court Judge Haynes was postponed for two days because of the death of a family member of one of the state's final witnesses.

April 5, 2005: Brian Lapps [Ex Director of Tenn Care] told the Senate Reform Committee [with his presentation titled: "The Truth: Clarification of Issues and Perspectives"] that Tenn Care "cannot be fixed without massive removal". Mr. Lapps further stated that he was displeased with State Officials and the Tennessee News Media for "not doing more to stem fraud in Tenn Care".

April 23, 2005: Governor Bredesen reassured that 323,000 adults that will lose Tenn Care will "receive adequate coverage through the state's safety net".

US District Court Hearing concerning of Tenn Care proposed cuts was delayed so that Federal Medicaid Officials have time to rule on the acceptability of the proposed changes by Tennessee.

April to May 2005: The following ocurred:

1. April 25, 2005: Opposition Groups broadcasted ads [in the media] defending Tenn Care against Cuts.

2. April 26, 2005: Governor Bredesen announced a deal that would protect 100,000 of the sickest against cuts.

3. April 29, 2005: Enrollment ends for some Tenn Care Programs.

4. May 17, 2005: The US Federal Government files a brief in favor of Tenn Care Cuts. AARP [American Association of Retired People] files a brief objecting to cuts.

5. May 22, 2005: The Office of Inspector General in Tennessee is criticized for not convicting people of Tenn Care Fraud. [This is taking into account a 5 Million Dollar Budget, and 30 Arrests]. Lawmakers commented that the money could have been used for health care.

6. May 23, 2005: Governor Bredesen tells lawmakers not "to attach too many strings on a 100 Million Dollar Plan sparing 97,000 Tenn Care enrollees from proposed cuts".

7. May 30, 2005: Tennessee sends Tenn Care Disenrollment Notes to those who will be removed from Tenn Care. Spokespeople for Public Hospitals state that they will be "hit hardest".

June 6, 2005: US District Judge John Nixon sets a tentative hearing date for June 28, 2005 with regards to Tenn Care. This is taking into account when the US Federal Center for Medicare and Medicaid Services rules on other aspects of the State's Plan to reform Tenn Care.

June 2005: Since June 20, 2005, People protesting the Tenn Care Cuts started a Sit at the State Capitol Rotunda. They vowed to remain in the Rotunda until the Governor stops sending termination letters. Governor Bredesen offered to meet with the protesters in private. But the protesters wanted a public meeting. The protesters have received additional support when the leadership of the Southern Christian Leadership Conference joined the sit in. Governor Bredesen has also met with the protestors. No results at the present time.

Tenn Care is a story that will continue to play itself out for some time. It is not known at the time of this writing what will be the end results. The only suggestion that the author could make is to check the websites and addresses of the following institutions:

The Tennessean
1100 Broadway
Nashville Tennessee 37203
www.tennessean.com

Center on Budget and Policy Priorities
820 First Street NE Suite 510
Washington DC 20002
www.cbpp.org

NewsMax.com

Bureau of Tenn Care
729 Church Street
Nashville Tennessee 37247-6501
www.tennessee.gov

Tennessee Health Care Campaign
1103 Chapel Ave.
Nashville Tennessee 37206

WSMV TV News
5700 Knob Road
Nashville Tennessee 37209
www.wsmv.com

5

MAINE

DIRIGO: Latin for "I Direct", "I Guide", "I Lead". It is also the State Motto of Maine.

During the last decade [the 1990's], Maine has not escaped the national discussion of Health Care Reform. Directly or indirectly, the people of Maine have been affected by rising health care costs, increase in health insurance premiums, accompanied by rising prescription medication prices, and barriers to services.

Those who have to do with Health Care as an Issue [Legislature, Consumers, Business, Health Care Providers, and Insurers] have presented/promoted concepts with the intention of widening access to services and care that is comprehensive.

Dirigo Health [Health Program in Maine] is working with other protagonists in the Maine Health Care Industry to guide strategically in future health services investment. With the development of a state health plan, insurers and providers [for planning purposes] have agreed to a voluntary one year limit on cost growth and new construction that increase health costs and are costly.

The State Health Plan is to strengthen a review of proposals submitted for investments, technologies, and new services under the Certificate of Need Program.

A Certificate of Need [in Maine] is the following: When Providers seek to invest in capital improvements which costs over 2.4 Million Dollars [this is subject to change] and/or in new technology, [that will cost over 1.2 Million Dollars]. The Providers and/or Institutions must submit an application for a Certificate of Need Approval. The Certificate of Need is reinforced by the State Health Plan and by the Maine Quality Forum.

Other Agencies in Dirigo Health are:

1. Dirigo Choice

2. Maine Care

3. Maine Quality Forum

4. Maine RX Plus

5. Governor's Office of Health Policy and Finance

Dirigo Choice is an affordable comprehensive health plan that is offered to small businesses, self employed, and individuals. It includes wellness and prevention programs. When a business offers Dirigo Choice, there are the advantages of:

1. Ability to retain employees and recruits new employees by businesses is enhanced.

2. Greater Health and Financial Security for Employer and Employee.

3. Healthier and Productive Work Force

Dirigo Choice helps small businesses and employees with the following:

1. Competitive High Quality Health Care Coverage.

2. Discounts which helps employees in affording the program.

3. Health Plan Costs Predictability.

4. Employers can retain employees and recruit new ones.

5. Offer Wellness Programs.

6. 100% Coverage for Preventive Services.

7. Improvement of Work Force Productivity.

8. Reduction of absenteeism.

Dirigo Choice [Competitive]:

1. Competitive Price more affordable via discounts that are tied to family size and income.

2. Monthly Premium Discounts, Reductions on Deductibles/Out of Pocket Expenses for those under a certain amount of the Federal Poverty Level.

Dirigo Choice [Employee Sensitive]:

1. Voluntary for Employees.

2. Employees must offer Family Coverage but they can pay 60% of employee only costs.

3. Employers are provided with more choice in health care coverage to employees.

Dirigo Choice [Prevention]:

1. History and Physical Examination, Blood Testing, Mammogram, Well Baby Care with 100% Coverage.

2. Discount at Fitness Clubs.

3. Healthy Maine Rewards Program: Members receive $100.00 Cash for meeting Health Goals.

Dirigo Choice [Comprehensive]: Hospital, Physician Visits, Prescription Medication Coverage.

Maine Care is the Medicaid Program [in Maine] with a combination of state and Federal [USA] Revenues. Services are provided to children, childless adults, families, senior citizens, and the disabled. Eligibility may vary between group and service types. It may also be based on household income and assets.

Maine Rx Plus is an agency that provides discounts on prescription medications for those who lack prescription coverage.

Maine Quality Forum [another part of Dirigo Health] whose purpose is to aim for high quality health care and help citizens of Maine make informed choices about their health care. They use the definition of High Quality Health Care defined by the Institute of Medicine [in its report "Crossing the Quality Chasm" from the year 2001]. The key tasks are the following:

1. Assess Medical Technology Needs throughout Maine.

2. Inform Certificate of Need Processes.

3. Collect Research on Quality of Health Care; Evidence Based Medicine, and Patient Safety.

4. Promote Use of best medical practices.

5. Coordinate efficient collection of health care data which would be used to assess the health care environment, facilitate improvement of quality, and consumer choice.

6. Promotion of Healthy Lifestyles.

7. Promotion of Safe and Efficient Care via Electronic Administration and Data Reporting.

Governor's Office of Health Policy and Finance [GOHPF]: has overall responsibility for the Dirigo Health Reform Act and is a liaison with the Dirigo Health Agency. GOHPF had to do with the development of Dirigo Health Reform Act. GOHPF directs policies pertaining to health care from the Governor's Office.

HISTORY OF THE DIRIGO HEALTH PROGRAM:
2002: John I. Baldacci [Democrat] is elected Governor of Maine on [partly] a platform of addressing cost, quality, and access to health care.

January 9, 2003: After his inauguration, Governor Baldacci signed an Executive Order which gave birth to the Governor's Office of Health Care Policy and Finance [GOHPF]. The purpose of GOHPF is to direct efforts in the reformation of health care. Governor Baldacci also establishes the Health Action Team [HAT]. HAT is a diverse group of stakeholders whose purpose is to advise the Governor and GOHPF.

March 5, 2003: Governor Baldacci [with GOHPF] announced a prescription medication plan for Great Northern Paper Company Workers and Retirees that are enrolled in the Health Coverage Program. Under this plan, participants are eligible for benefits of up to $58.00 per prescription after a $10.00 co payment. This will include the amount in which a prescription price may exceed $1000.00. If an Eligible Plan Participant uses a Network Pharmacy, he/she will not be required to pay more than $932.00 + applicable $10.00. Participants are eligible [if they use limited Out of Network Services] for Benefits of Up to $29.00 per prescription.

May 5, 2003: Governor Baldacci presented the Dirigo Health Reform Initiative. This represented a reform of Maine's Health Care System in a comprehensive way. The reform included measures designed to control the growth of health care costs, ensure statewide quality of care, with access to affordable quality coverage. Certain stakeholders expressed concerns about key areas of the initiative. GOHPF and the Stakeholders discussed these [concerns] with the Governor and the Joint Select Committee on Health Care Reform [Maine State Legislature].

May 19, 2003: The Maine Supreme Court lifted an injunction of the District Court in Maine RX Case. [It must be worth remembering that there was a prescription program called Healthy Maine Prescription Programs which was started in June 2001 and was ordered discontinued in December 2002 by a Federal Circuit Court].

May 30, 2003: Governor Baldacci presented a new prescription medication benefit called Maine RX Plus. Maine RX Plus provided greater discounts than the previous benefit plan [See May 19, 2003]. Maine RX Plus was to be included in Dirigo Health. In a Press Conference, Governor Baldacci stated that Maine RX Plus complements the Dirigo Health Plan by improving the quality of health care [by providing access to lower priced medications].

June 18, 2003: Dirigo Health is signed by Governor Baldacci as a Law.

September 5, 2003: Governor Baldacci appoints five voting members and three non voting members to the Dirigo Health Board of Directors.

October 9, 2003: Governor Baldacci announced a 9 person hospital commission which would work with GOHPF, report on hospital costs and services. This hospital commission would make recommendations which would strengthen and rationalize the delivery of hospital services in Maine.

November 3, 2003: Governor Baldacci swore in the Board of Directors for Dirigo Health. He also received the American Public Health Association [APHA] Distinguished Public Health Legislator of the Year Award for his "leadership in the establishment of the Dirigo Health Plan".

November 7, 2003: Appointments to the Task Force on Veterans Health Services were announced by the Governor. The Purpose of the Task Force is to analyze and assess Health Services to Veterans, Work Closely with the [US] Federal Government and make recommendations in order to effectively organize veteran services.

December 22, 2003: Information from the State Bureau of Insurance was released to the people of Maine. This information shows the slowing of growth rate insurance premiums in 2003. The Governor stated that he was pleased with the results, yet more should be done "to create and maintain lower health costs".

January 9, 2004: Thomas J. Dunne appointed the First Executive Director of Dirigo Health by the Governor and the Chief of Board of Directors of the Dirigo Health Agency; Robert Mc Afee.

January 27, 2004: Governor Baldacci announces that the State of Maine will provide a brochure to help residents control health care costs by giving residents the tools to compare hospital and health care center prices.

February 13, 2004: The Governor announced the availability of a new brochure on the Dirigo Health Reform Act. This brochure is to provide an overview of the reform act and place emphasis on cost, quality, and access.

March 12, 2004: Dr. Dennis Shubert is selected by the Dirigo Health Agency Executive Director and the Governor to head the Maine Quality Forum.

April 28, 2004: Governor Baldacci announces an initiative to assist Medicare Beneficiaries in accessing Prescription Discount Cards.

May 7, 2004: Governor Baldacci announced that Dirigo Health Policy will release a RFP [Request for Proposal] to seek bids from Insurance Companies with the intent of carrying the Dirigo Health Plan.

May 13, 2004: Dirigo Health Reform receives a major grant of $887,133 from the Maine Health Access Foundation [MeHAF]

May 13, 2004 [Part II]: The funds for MeHAF Grant are to be used to support the following activities:

1. Development of a Comprehensive Health Plan which will ensure access to care that is affordable and of high quality.

2. Commission for studying Maine's Hospitals which will engage in intensive reviews of Maine's Hospital with the purpose of presenting a final report.

3. Marketing of the Dirigo Health Plan.

The Administrative and Logistic Support for the grant will be by NASHP [National Academy for State Health Policy].

Before continuing, let us define Me HAF and NASHP.

Me HAF is a foundation that was established in April 2000 after the sale of Blue Cross/Blue Shield of Maine to Anthem Insurance Company. It is the largest non-profit health care foundation in Maine that supports strategic solutions in addressing the health care needs in Maine [with emphasis on the uninsured.]

NASHP is a nonprofit organization based in Portland Maine. It works with states across the USA to support their efforts in the improvement of health care quality and access.

June 11, 2004: Anthem Blue Cross/Blue Shield of Maine submitted a bid with the intention of partnering with the Dirigo Health Agency in the administration of the Dirigo Health Plan.

July 26, 2004: GOHPF [Governor's Office of Health Policy and Finance] released a one year State Plan [which will be transitional until the first biennial state plan goes into effect on July 1, 2005].
The key objective of this provisional plan included the following:

1. Reduction of the number of Uninsured Maine Residents by 31,000.

2. Set priorities and target spending for new investments in health care facilities and equipment.

3. Reduction of inappropriate use of hospital emergency departments by mental health patients accompanied by development of preventive and community options.

4. Development of Specific Strategies that would reduce the amount of chronic illness.

5. Ensure that Maine Residents receive the best practices in Medical Care.

6. Simplification of Billing Practices.

7. Initiate Payment Methods that reward good performance.

8. Engage Citizens in the discussion of Health Care Priorities.

July 27, 2004: GOHPF issued Emergency Rules for the establishment of the Capital Investment Funds [CIF] as a response to business leaders, consumers, one of the major hospital systems. CIF was established after it was determined that Health Care Costs in Maine were increasing more than the income of a Maine Citizen.

According to a GOHPF Report: "Between 1996 and 2002, the cost of a family policy for Maine Businesses and Employees increased by 77%, median income increased by 6% and increase for small businesses are steeper"

August 6, 2004: GOHPF released CIF. Before hospitals/health care providers could spend on facilities, equipments, and services that are potentially costly, A Certificate of Need IS Necessary.

August 16, 2004: GOHPF announces an ad campaign and a new website with the purpose of increasing awareness of Maine Residents of Dirigo Health Reform and Care.

August 23, 2004: Anthem Blue Cross/Blue Shield of Maine reached an agreement with the State of Maine concerning the administration of Dirigo Choice. Thomas Dunne resigns as Executive Director of the Dirigo Health Agency.

Sept. 7, 2004: Karynlee Harrington is named New Executive Director of the Dirigo Health Agency.

September 13, 2004: First Anniversary of Dirigo Health becoming law. The Governor also announced that Dirigo Choice will be launched with Anthem Blue Cross/Blue Shield. Marketing is targeted to begin October 1, 2004. Enrollment is targeted to begin January 1, 2005.

November 5, 2004: The website for Maine Quality Forum is launched.

December 22, 2004: The Commission to study Maine's Hospitals released a draft report with recommendations for affordable, accessible, quality hospital care. Report to be finalized in January 2005

January 3, 2005: Dirigo Choice Coverage celebrated by businesses in Maine.

January 10, 2005: Maine Care Fact Book released by GOHPF

February 2, 2005: Final Report by the Commission to Study Maine's Hospital Released.

March 11, 2005: WLBZ 2 [A Television Station in Maine] reported on a Video Conference which was a product of the GOHPF. The video conference was to connect 1000 Maine Residents for a discussion on Health Care. Residents participating in this discussion were to be asked about their opinions with regards to regulating hospitals, health care providers with the intention of limiting costs. GOHPF announced that the input was to be used to develop the biennial health plan. Opponents stated that "the conference was a waste of time and can be used for political capital for Governor Baldacci and Dirigo Health." The Maine Hospital Association stated that members agreed on "voluntary caps on cost increases and margins of operations."

March 15, 2005: Republican Lawmakers held a News Conference on the Maine State House. The purpose was to offer "alternatives to the Health Insurance Crisis". Republican Legislators criticized "mandated coverage provisions of Dirigo Health since Health Insurance Markets could be distorted."

March 15, 2005: The Health Insurance Companies VS GOHPF: In response to a proposal by opponents of the Dirigo Health Care Plan to create a high risk pool and eliminate guaranteed issue were met with a response to a study by the GOHPF comparing Maine's Program to New Hampshire and Kentucky.

According to the GOHPF [Maine] Study:
"New Hampshire: initiated High Risk Pool in the summer of 2002. Around the End of 2003, 158 People out of the total population of New Hampshire [1.3 Million] were enrolled. March 2005: Premiums were $1375 Per Month for Oldest Smoking Members. Maternity Riders [which are optional] were an additional $432 to $851 a month.

Kentucky: Started Enrollment on January 1, 2001. By the end of 2003, 2457 OF Kentucky's 4.1 Million People were enrolled. March 2005: Premiums were as high as $872 per month for men over age 65. Mental Health/Substance Abuse/ Pharmacy Riders [depending on age and gender] were $80 to $500 a month.

Percentage of uninsured in New Hampshire and Kentucky increased in 2001, 2002, 2003.

Maine: Dirigo Choice is expanding health care access. Inappropriate Utilization and High Costs of Services are being addressed by the State Health Plan, Certificate of Need Program, and Capital Investment Plan. Maine remains a leader in pharmaceutical cost containment. High Rates of Costly Chronic Conditions are addressed.

April 1, 2005: According to GOHPF, Dirigo Choice continues to have strong enrollment.

May 2, 2005: The Governor [with Senator Michael Brenman, hospital representatives, parents, children, family advocates] announced that Dirigo Choice is "helping more families have access to quality, affordable, and accessible health care and insurance."

The saga continues.....

6

KENTUCKY

The GOHPF [Maine] Report commented on High Risk Pools in Kentucky and New Hampshire. In the year 2004, Kentucky embarked on Health Care Reform.

In 2004, Ernie Fletcher [Republican] took the oath of office as Governor of Kentucky. He stated in his innaugural speech about the need to "Move Forward". At this time, Kentucky was running a deficit with its Medicaid Program.

Kentucky's Medicaid System was costly, insuficient, and unable to satisfy the needs of its subscribers. Kentucky was one of least healthy states with an incidence of obesity [6th place] and diabetes [7th place]. Kentucky was also in the high rankings in deaths due to cancer and/or cardiovascular disease. Kentucky's Medicaid Program was 22% of the Annual Expenditures. 11.4% of Kentucky's State General Funds were spent in Medicaid. Kentucky's Medicaid Program had an annual budget of 4.7 Billion Dollars with a 675 Million Short Fall in FY 2006. Remember, Kentucky's Medicaid Program covers more than 691,000 enrollees at the time of this article.

Kentucky had ranked 47% in the nation for median household [$34,368 compared to the national median income of $43,564]. The Poverty Level in Kentucky was worse than the national level.

The Medicaid Program in Kentucky was in need of a major restructuring.

The background was laid for Ky Health Choices. Ky Health Choices [Kentucky Health Choices] is an improved Medicaid Program.

The goals were twofold:

1. Address the Needs of the Subscriber Population.

2. Encourage Personal Involvement on the part of the subscriber population in their health care.

The Subscriber Population may be enrolled in one of the four available health plans:

1. Global Choices

2. Family Choices

3. Optimum Choices

4. Comprehensive Choices

Global Choices is the overall Medicaid Program.

Family Choices will cover the KCHIP [Kentucky Children's Health Insurance Program] and most children. KCHIP was established in 1999 with the mission of providing health insurance to uninsured children who come from low income families.

Optimum Choices covers individuals who are in need of long term care treatment and/or those who suffer from mental impairment.

Comprehensive Choices deals with acquired brain injuries, nursing home facility levels, and the geriatric age bracket.

Under Ky Health Choices, Medicaid automatically signs the potential subscriber. The subscriber retains his/her cureent Medicaid Card.

The subscriber will have services limited in scopes [classified as soft limits]. He/She will not lose any services. Prescription Medications will be limited to four medications per month.

If a subscriber is in need of more services secondary to health related issues [including pharmaceuticals], the limit will be waived. The Health Care Professional should document justifications as to why limits should be waived.

The following diseases were exonerated from the limits:

1. Hypertension

2. Type II Diabetes Mellitus

3. Alzheimer's Dementia

4. Cancer

5. Lung Cancer

6. End Stage Renal Disease

7. Hypercholesterolemia

8. Metabolic Syndrome

9. Terminal Phase of an Illness

10. Hemophilia

11. HIV/AIDS

12. Cystic Fibrosis

13. Migraine Headaches

14. Organ Transplant

15. Epilepsy

16. Thyroid Cancer

17. Heart Disease

There is a country song titled: "Rose Garden". One of it verse states the following: "I Never Promised You a Rose Garden". The song can be applied to Ky Health Choices because the best things in life are NOT FREE.

There is a co-payment for certain services which could range between One Dollar to Ten Dollars. Each service will have a table corresponding to the co-payments. The Co-Payments will vary with the service.

THERE ARE NO CO-PAYMENTS ON PREVENTIVE SERVICE SINCE ONE OF THE PURPOSES OF KY HEALTH CHOICES IS TO MAKE THE SUBSCRIBER THE PROTAGONIST OF HIS/HER HEALTH.

Ky Health Choices has an initiative called Get Healthy Accounts. The subscriber can receive awards for maintaining appointments or refilling medications in a timely manner. These rewards can be used for membership in a gymnasium, weight loss program, and smoking cessation program.

August 19, 2005: Kentucky signed a 5 year contract with First Health Services with the purpose of administering Ky Health Services. [First Health Services also has a contract with Kentucky's Pharmacy Based Administrator [PBA]. [There is another contract in existence between EDS and MMIS: Medicaid Management Information System].

First Health Services was assigned to administer the policies and guidelines of DMS [Kentucky Department of Medical Services] which is related to provider/member education, case management, and disease management.

Ky Health Choices was to coordinate a new credentialing process for provider [based on practices in the private sector with peer review organization and a full serviced call center].

December 2005: Governor Ernie Fletcher appoints Mark D. Birdwhistell as Secretary of State of Kentucky's Cabinet for Health and Family Services.

January 2006: Kentucky launched a self funded health plan for state government employees [active and/or retired]. This plan is to be administered by a third party policy administrator. With this, the Commonwealth of Kentucky can focus on program design, consistency, stability, and/or predictability.

January 18, 2006: Ky Health Choices received Federal Approval for Medicaid Report.

February 1, 2006: Governor Ernie Fletcher announced [and was reported on WAVE 3 TV] his goals for reshaping Kentucky Medicaid. The goals were to reduce costs without sacrificing health care.

February-March 2006: Medicaid Commissioner Shannon Turner expressed hope for a "seamless transition" with a gradual phasing in of the program.

Since Ky Health Choices is in its infancy, it would be best to do more detailed studies in the future with the purpose of rating it objectively.

Readers could visit the Commonwealth of Kentucky Website at kentucky.gov and/or WAVE 3 at www.wave3.com

WAVE 3 TV
725 S Floyd St
Louisville KY 40203

7

WISCONSIN

Wisconsin [like most states] began the journey towards Health Care Reform in the 1990's. During this period, Governor Tommy Thompson [Republican] proposed a Health Care Plan which was to replace Medicaid. This was to take into account low income working families that were making the transition from Welfare to Work Force.

1997: Wisconsin submits a waiver proposal to the US Federal Government with the intention of covering low income adults with children using funds from Medicaid.

August 1998: The [US] Federal Government denies the waiver because of inclusion of adults.

January 1999: CMS [The Center for Medicare Medicaid Services] formerly HCFA [Health Care Finance Administration] [USA] granted Wisconsin a Regular Medicaid Waiver which allowed enrollment of parents who were earning below 185% of the Federal Poverty Level.

July 1999: Badger Care begins enrollment with less than 8,647 people initially. February 2005: Badger Care Enrollment is more than 91,000. [See Graphs and Power Point Slides in next pages]

HISTORICAL	BADGER CARE	ENROLLMENT
Jul-99	4,728	SERIES 1
Jul-00	41,380	SERIES 2
Jul-01	73,843	SERIES 3
Jul-02	89,119	SERIES 4

Jul-03	112,776	SERIES 5
Jul-04	131,433	SERIES 6
Feb-05	135,561	SERIES 7

Reference: State of Wisconsin Department of Health and Family Services: February 2005

BADGER CARE	ENROLLMENT	BY CATEGORY	Feb-05	
ENROLLEES	150% FPL	>150% FPL	TOTAL	%
CHILDREN	22,715	6,854	29,569	-2.42%
PARENTS	53,480	8,223	61,703	-1.63%
TOTAL	76,195	15,077	91,272	-1.89%

Reference: State of Wisconsin Department of Health and Family Services: February 2005

CHILDREN	ENROLLLED	IN MEDICAID DUE TO	BADGER CARE
Jan-05	106,970		
Feb-05	105,992		
NET CHA	-978		
% CHANGE	-0.91		

Reference: State of Wisconsin Department of Health and Family Services: February 2005

Reference: State of Wisconsin Department of Health and Family Services: February 2005

WISCONSIN BADGER CARE FUNDING & ENROLLMENT WITH TITLE XXI WAIVER

BUDGETED	ENROLLMENT		
	SFY 2005	SFY 2006	SFY 2007
CHILDREN	44,806	30,603	31,849
PARENTS	81,008	63,359	65,940
TOTAL	125,814	93,961	97,789

Reference: State of Wisconsin Department of Health and Family Services: February 2005

WISCONSIN BADGER CARE FUNDING & ENROLLMENT WITH TITLE XXI WAIVER

STATE FISCAL	YEAR BUDGET		
	SFY 2005	SFY 2006	SFY 2007
STATE	68,401,100	64,204,720	76,688,100
FEDER	139,339,500	120,880,500	130,153,000
PR.REV	8,954,300	7,011,000	7,439,500
TOTAL	216,754,900	192,096,220	214,280,600

Reference: State of Wisconsin Department of Health and Family Services: February 2005

Badger Care:
Definition: Health Insurance Program of Wisconsin

Purpose: For Working Families with Children. It provides coverage to those families whose incomes are too high for Medicaid yet there is no access for health care.

Goal:

1. Elimination of barriers to [successful] employment by providing a transition from welfare to private insurance.

2. It is based on the following premise: "Health Care is Essential for Working Families with Children".

Basic Provisions:

1. Low Income Families that are not eligible for Medicaid can qualify for Badger Care if their income is below 185% of the Federal Poverty Level. [Everything changes when the threshold of 200% Federal Poverty Level is reached].

2. No Asset or Means Test Required.

3. Patients with insurance in the past three months [including group insurance paid by the employer [80%] is ineligible.

4. Most Recipients are enrolled in a Managed Care Setting.

Funding and Operating Authority: Badger Care Funding is limited to amounts destined for the program. If costs exceed budgeted levels, Wisconsin has the authority to impose an "enrollment trigger" [which is subject to approval by the Joint Committee on Finance] which would reduce income levels at which new families may enroll.

[It must be taken into account that Title XIX Enrollment Trigger may be used to increase or decrease the income level for eligibility on an initial basis. This may lead to loss of Federal Matching Rates for Parents.]

Regardless, adjustments had to be made. On February 3 2004, Ms. Helene Nelson [Secretary of the State of Wisconsin Department of Health and Family Services] wrote a letter to the Friends of Public Health asking the DHFS [Department of Health and Family Services] for help in the development of recommendations meant to improve the Public Health System by:

1. Streamlining State Government.

2. Elimination of Redundant Work in Public Health.

3. Increasing resources available in the community for effective public health.

4. Check alternative forms for funding.

5. Improve the capacity for Wisconsin to carry on its mission of public health and achieve the goals set by Healthiest Wisconsin 2010.

On November 30, 2004, CBS 5 WFRV [One of the TV Stations in Wisconsin] had a program related to consumer directed health care. It dealt with an alternative in health care in which the mindset of entitlement is replaced by Consumer directed Health Care. Under this approach, the consumer would be directly responsible for how they spend their money for health care. It would be followed by Cost Awareness and Ownership. The participants agreed on the need to educate consumers so that they could learn how to be responsible for their health care.

The 2005-2007 Biennial Budget of the Governor of Wisconsin includes the following for the Department of Health and Family Services. [It would be worth while to check the website].

I. Budget Priorities set by the Governor:

1. Balanced Budget without tax increase.

2. Streamlining of State Government Operations.

3. Supporting Healthy/Safe Kids and Strong Families with the implementation of Kids First.

4. Preserve Access to Health Care.

5. Increasing Patient Safety and Reducing Health Care Costs via initiatives pertaining to health care quality and medical technology.

The General Over view is the Preservation of the Health Care Safety Net [Medical Assistance, Badger Care, and Senior Care]:

1. Measures which control costs and maximizes revenue from the US Federal Government.

2. No Reduction of eligibility and service coverage.

3. No Increase in Client Cost Sharing.

Income Maintenance:

I. Medical Assistance Quality Assurance:

1. Implementation of State QA Reviews with the intention of monitoring trends, errors, and determining etiology of errors.

2. Implementation of Local Second Party Review.

3. Provision of technical assistance and training with the purpose of implementing corrective action.

4. Increasing Data Revenue for Eligibility Verification.

II. Changing the Medicaid Grace Month:

1. Purpose is to terminate eligibility at the end of the 12 Month Period [in order to establish a consistency with the US Federal Regulations].

III. Recovery of Incorrect Badger Care and Medicaid Payments:

Income Maintenance:
III. Recovery of Incorrect Badger Care and Medicaid Payments:

1. Increase of $70,000 in SFY 2007 which would reflect an increase in revenue from allowing DHFS to recover overpayments which are a result of failure in reporting changes in non financial criteria [change in residency, household consumption or Insurance Coverage for Badger Care]

2. Statutory Language Changes which would allow DHFS to expedite process of acquiring court orders with the intention of allowing recoveries to be made through the use of tax interceptions.

Medical Assistance:
I. Badger Care Re-estimates:
Decrease of $287 Million in all funds during the biennium of 2005-2007 which has been due to a decrease in enrollment in FY 2005 [Caseload in FY 2004 =113,000 To FY 2005 = 94,473].
This is the Expected resumption of Growth after FY 2005. [This is the Projected Growth in FY 2006 = 92,301 and FY 2007 = 96,022].

II. Expansion of SSI [Supplemental Security Income] Managed Care *: [SSI= Supplemental Security Income: Federal Government Income Support Program] for the aged, blind, and disabled.]

1. Phase-in in Milwaukee in April to June 2005 followed by further expansion into La Crosse County, and Southeast Wisconsin for FY 2006.

III. Wisconsin Medicaid Cost Reporting:

1. To be continued on an ongoing basis.

2. Increase in 13.2% in FY 2006 and Maintenance of this level in FY 2007.

3. Generates Net Savings of $20 Million in the 2005-2007 Program in Medical Assistance.

IV. Medicaid HMO Provider Assessment and Rate Increase:

1. Establishment of a 6% Provider Agreement on Gross Revenues on licensed HMOS that serve Medicaid Recipients.

2. 7.6% Rate Increase for HMO'S in 2005-2007 Period.

Medical Assistance:

IV. Medicaid HMO Provider Assessment and Rate Increase:

3. Assessment would affect HMOs serving Medicaid and Badger Care Patients.

4. The effects of these changes are a net savings of $42,528,200 in the 2005-2007 Period.

V. Medicaid, Badger Care, and Senior Care Pharmacy Reimbursements:

1. Redirection of Pharmacy Reimbursements for Brand Name Medication from the average wholesale price minus 13% to minus 16%.

2. Elimination of Senior Care 5% Enhancement for Brand Name Medications.

3. Reduction of dispensing Fee from $4.38 to $3.88 per prescription.

4. Provide savings of $7,272,000 GPR [General Purpose Revenue] [$9,094,800 Federal] for Fiscal Year 2006 and $10,559,700 [$13,880,400 Federal] in Fiscal Year 2007.

VI. Health Care Quality Improvement Fund:

1. Establishment of HCQI [Health Care Quality Improvement Fund with the intention of funding Medical Assistance Benefits.

2. Transfer of $179.4 Million of Funds from Patient Compensation into the HCQI Fund. [$150 Million of these funds will be used for Medical Assistance Base Benefits. $19.4 Million will fund MA Supplemental Hospital Payments]

Medical Assistance:

VI. Health Care Quality Improvement Fund:

3. Transfer of $130 Million of Funding from the State of Wisconsin Revenue Bonds into the HCQI which will be utilized to fund Medical Assistance Base Benefits.

Public Health:
Health Care Information:

1. Elimination of the Board of Health Care Information as of October 1, 2005 and its replacement with the Health Care Quality and Patient Safety Board [HCQPSB].

2. HCQPSB is to develop a plan with the intention of improving health care data technology. HCQPSB will be authorized to make grants and loans to entities with that purpose.

3. Transfer of $250,000 a year from DHFS Physician Assessment Revenue to a new Health Care Quality Improvement Fund with the intention of funding HCQPSB.

4. Transfer of $10 Million from Patient Compensation Fund to HCQI Fund with the purpose of Improvement in Health Care Information and Technology.

Governor Boyle also announced the creation of Badger Rx Gold with the intention of giving Wisconsin Residents an option in less expensive medications.

More can be mentioned about Health Care Changes in Wisconsin. Only Time will reveal whether the changes have or have not benefited Wisconsin.

For further information: Please visit the State of Wisconsin Website at http://www.dhfs.state.wi.us/badgercare/.

Also, please feel free to write to:
State of Wisconsin Secretary Department of Health and Family Services
1 West Wilson Street
Post Office Box 7850
Madison Wisconsin 53707-7850

WFRV TV 5 CBS
Health watch
Attn: Miss Lisa Malak
1181 East Mason Street
Green Bay Wisconsin 54301
www.wfrv.com

8

NEVADA

The year 2005 was one of Health Care Changes in Nevada. Examples of these changes are in the following Assembly Bills that have been proposed in the 73rd Legislative Session in Nevada.

March 10, 2005: State Assembly Majority Leader Barbara Buckley introduced Assembly Bill 195. She did this as a response to the increasing costs of prescription medication.

The purpose of Assembly Bill 195 is to require the State of Nevada Pharmacy Board to inspect and license pharmacies in Canada. This was to be followed by the creation of a website which would link Nevada Consumers to Canadian Pharmacies. When [and if this bill should pass], Nevada would be joining states [such as Minnesota] in importing pharmaceutical medications.

Other dates in Assembly Bill 195 worth mentioning:
March 10, 2005: It was read for the first time.
March 11, 2005: It was sent to Committee.
April 20, 2005: From the Committee [it was amended] and placed on the second reading file.
April 21, 2005: Passed by a 29 to 12 vote
April 22, 2005: In the Senate.

Other bills [such as AB296, AB322, and AB342] were passed by the Nevada Legislature. The Democrats labeled these [bills] as "Cost Containment Bills". Assembly Woman Sheila Leslie [Democrat-Reno] stated the following: "The more information we obtain, the better we can regulate....I hope that the information will help us arrive at the root cause of Nevadans having to pay the top hospital costs".

The response of Assembly Minority Leader Lynn Hetwick [Republican-Gardner-ville] objected by saying: "It will be costly reporting. I don't think reporting does much of anything."

AB296, AB322, and AB342 require hospitals with more than 100 beds to spend 4% of its profits in indigent care or investments in the community. It also requires that hospitals that are operated by Out of State [Non-Nevada] Corporations to file more detailed reports on earnings. There is an additional mandate: "All Major Hospitals must give patients more information on pricing."

SB9 is another bill that was introduced by the Department of Human Resources and Education. The purpose of is to increase the amount in which certain hospitals are required to reduce or discount certain charges billed to uninsured patients and those eligible for Medicare.
February 7, 2005: SB 9 was read and sent to committee
April 16, 2005: No further action was allowed on SB9.

May 12, 2005: The US Federal Government announced the setting aside of a billion dollars [nationally] with the purpose of treating illegal immigrants in states like California, Nevada, and Texas. Nevada is to receive 24 Million Dollars. With this news, hospitals that treat illegal immigrants can now bill the Federal Government. Miguel Barrientos [of Southwest Hispanic Media] states: "We don't want the American Public to think that their taxes are paying for illegals to receive treatment. It is not true. This is their money going back for health care." Anne Lynch of Sunrise Hospital in Las Vegas Nevada stated: "Two Million Dollars for Nevada is not a swipe at the uninsured."

Still, the situation for Nevada is only the beginning. It would be wise to check the following sites:
State of Nevada State Legislature: www.leg.state.nv.us

KLAS TV 8 Newsroom
3228 Channel 8 Dr.
Las Vegas Nevada 89109
www.klas-tv.com

9

MISCELLANEOUS INFORMATION

According to reports from KOB TV 4 [NBC Affiliate in New Mexico], The University of New Mexico will be eliminating its hospice program for adults by July 1 2005. They will leave the Pediatric Hospice Program intact. [The population of the Pediatric Hospice Program is 0]. Hospital Spokeswoman Ms. Jennifer Riordan states that "the 27 patients currently in hospice will continue to receive care until they die but new patients will be referred to other hospices." Ms. Riordan states that the closures were for "financial reasons and that the hospital [University of New Mexico] could save $250,000 to $500,000 a year".

Advocates for poor patients have been commenting about the denial of health care for the poor in the University of New Mexico Hospital [located in Albuquerque New Mexico]. The response of Steve Mc Kernan [CEO of the University of New Mexico Hospital in Albuquerque] was that "poor patients are getting the care needed but that the number of people without health insurance is growing."

The Indian Hospital in Albuquerque New Mexico [and the Santa Clara Pueblo Clinic] has also been affected by reduction of services. Native Americans have been seeking alternative services at the Santa Fe Indian Hospital.

There have been recent news stories from Canada, Germany, and Great Britain which talks about changes in places where National Health Insurance is a reality.

Before talking about Canada, it should be remembered that its National Health System originated from a Decentralized Framework. It started when Saskatchewan introduced its Universal Health Insurance Program in 1946. By 1961, other Canadian Provinces introduced their Universal Health Insurance

Programs. In 1966, the Medical Care Act was passed by Canada's Parliament. [The Medical Care Act of Canada 1966 [Medicare] was 8 pages in comaprison with 35,000 pages in statutes, regulations, and manuals governing Medicare in the USA].In 1984, the Canada Health Act was passed by Parliament to end "extra billing". ["Extra Billing" was the additional fees on patients for services.

Yet in Canada, [secondary to the economic situations] there have been reductions in Federal Government Contributions to Health Care.

In June of 2005, the Supreme Court of Canada ruled in favor of those in Quebec who wanted to pay for Health Care Procedures covered by Medicare. This ruling affected the policy of Quebec's Health Care System against private payments for Medicare Covered Procedures. [Quebec's Charter does not guarantee a Constitutional Right to Health Care]

This ruling was not without its critics. Ms. Mary Boyd: [Chairperson of the Prince Edward Island Health Coalition] expressed fears that such a ruling could "alter the balance of health care delivery". The Quebec Government announced its intention to apply for a stay [between 6 months to 2 years] for the Court Decision to take effect.

There were demonstrations by Quebec Nurses against the Supreme Court Ruling. Michele Brisclair [Vice President of the Quebec Federation of Nurses] stated that "A Private Health Care System will not reduce waiting lists in the public sector". Michele Brisclair also asked Quebec Premier Jean Charest [Parti Quebecois] to "use his powers to overrule the Supreme Court Decision".

Germany now has an alternative in its Universal Health Care System with one condition. Under the German Plan, an individual can change from utilizing the Government Health Care to a Private One [but such a person CANNOT return to the Government Plan after leaving it].

Great Britain [known for its National Health Service] has also had its share of problems.

A BBC News article titled: "Fire Crews Replacing Paramedics" [dated July 31, 2002] commented about the use of Fire Services in Medical Emergencies where there is a lack of existence in Ambulances.

In the year 2004, the Health Care Commission Inspection Body announced BBC Spotlight [a Regional TV News Program] from BBC Southwest reported [by Health Correspondent Ms. Sally Mc Namara on April 14, 2005] on the death of a blind patient who was carrying MRSA [Methicillin Resistant Staphylococcus Aureus]. The Widow of the patient blamed Government Targets and announced a lawsuit against the hospital. Ms. Judith Jolly [A Liberal Democratic Party MP for Plymouth] commented that "hospitals should concentrate on patient care and not on targets."

May 13, 2005: During the Alan Beswick Show, [a radio program on BBC GMR heard regularly by the underwriter on Real Player], the Community Health Counsellor and Private Pension Representative of North Manchester Hospital commented on the "use of the private sector to alleviate pressure points in the Medical System".

May 24, 2005: In another news release from BBC, 14 acres from St Michael's Hospital in Aylsham were offered for sale.

May 27, 2005: BBC Midlands Today [in their story "NHS and Pacemaker] commented about a patient who was not paid by NHS for a Pacemaker. In the end, he went to Northamptonshire [where the NHS could pay for his pacemaker].

Again, only time will tell how Medicine may evolve in Canada, Germany, and Great Britain.

More Information can be obtained from:

BBC GMR
PO Box 951
Oxford Road
Manchester M60 1SD England Great Britain

Spotlight
BBC South West
Broadcasting House
Seymour Road
Plymouth
PL3 5BD England Great Britain

BBC Midlands Today
The Mailbox
Birmingham
B1 1RF England Great Britain

Canadian Broadcasting Corporation
P.O. Box 500 Station A
Toronto, ON M5W 1E6
Canada

Radio Canada International
1400, boulevard René-Lévesque Est
Montreal, QC
Canada
H2L 2M2

KOB-TV News Assignment Desk
4 Broadcast Plaza SW
Albuquerque, NM 87104

10

EPILOGUE

In this book, the underwriter did an in depth research of 6 states [Oregon, Minnesota, Tennesee, Maine, Wisconsin, and Nevada] and did some other researches of other states and countries [on a lesser scale].

With the exception of Maine, the underwriter was unable to appreciate the presence of health care as a right in the statutes of other states. Regardless, Chandler Woodcock (Campaigning for the Republican Nomination as Governor of Maine) proposed a Health Care Reform which would have "less government regulation, mor promotion of wellness programs, and a big dose of Medicaid Reform". Oregon is pushing for an initiative [and referendum] on making Health Care as a right for the 2006 election. Also in Oregon, the 9th US Circuit of Appeals ruled that "Elderly and Disabled People cut by the Oregon Legislature from the Oregon Health Plan [in 2003] can sue the state for Nursing Home Care. Dr. Allen Douma was selected by the State of Oregon, on March 12, 2006 to lead the Oregon Health Plan. Dr. Douma stated that he "hopes to develop partnerships between public agencies and health care providers to make health care more efficient. Minnesota is debating a bill that would require health insurance by 2007.

The underwriter wants to encourage a public discussion of health care. This discussion is necessary in an era of the Baby Boom Generation entering the 60's age range. It is also necessary in the discussion to consider those who cannot afford to pay for their health care secondary to job loss, and or homelessness.

[The underwriter was driving in a busy intersection. In this intersection, he saw an individual dressed in suit and tie. He was asking for money to pay for

his son's treatment in a hospital. His employment as well as his Health Insurance had been terminated.]

This book was not intended as a cure all for all of the problems facing Health Care. The underwriter was addressing the past and the present in Health Care & Reform in that realm.

It is of the opinion of the underwriter that the solutions [which are not easy] have to be initiated by the governing bodies and the general public. For a start, the concept of one size fits all mentality in Medicine will have to go. States and Individuals have to work on this problem on a one to one basis.

Politicians should work [for the general public] in making sure that there is a mechanism of Checks, and Balances, [with a transparent process of accountability] when it comes to Health Care Alloted Money.

The General Public should [and must] educate themselves about the choices that exist in Health Care. This would include medical treatment, cost of treatment, cost effectiveness of treatment, and if treatment is medically necessary.

Health Insurance Companies should also work with the politicians and the General Public in finding solutions to the Health Care Situation.

It should be remembered that the past is past, the present is here, and the future is molded by what is reaped and sown today.

REFERENCE

◆

[ASSESSED BY THE UNDERWRITER FROM FEBRUARY 2005 TO 2006]

1. "Rationing" Microsoft Encarta Online Encyclopedia 2004. http://encarta.msn.com. 1997-2004.

2. "Rationing: 'only option' for NHS" BBC News 2003. http://news.bbc.co.uk/1/hi/health/1156665.stm

3. "Healthy Policy for Low Income People in Oregon" Sparer, Michael S. Urban Institute. Sept. 24, 1999 http://www.urban.org/ur/print.cfm?

4. http://www.dhs.state.or.us/aboutdhs/overview.html 2004

5. ""11/2003" Oregon Health Plan Comparison Charts" Oregon Health Plan, State of Oregon DHS 2003.

6. "Oregon Health Plan: "Standard" and "Plus"". www.dhs.state.or.us/healthplan/app_benefits/standard_plus.html. State of Oregon DHS OHP 2004

7. "Client Handbook for the Oregon Health Plan". Oregon Health Plan, Office of Medical Assistance Program, Department of Human Services, July 2003. pgs. 27, 50 to 57.

8. "2003-2005 Legislative Session: Major Initiatives and the 2003-2005 Budget" Oregon Department of Human Services page 3.

9. "Oregon "Health Care Rationing" Plan: Bad Idea for Minnesota Patients; Citizens' Council on Health Care, http://www.cchc-mn.org/issues/against_healthplan.php2004

10. arcweb.sos.state.or.us/banners/governors.htm

11. www.omip.state.or.us/

12. www.ipgb.state.or.us/fhiap/index.html

13. egov.oregon.gov/DHS/NEWS/MESSAGE/news/2004_05_28.shtml.

14. "Power to the People: Positive Alternatives to the Oregon Health Plan". Ferrara, Peter J. Cascade Policy Institue October 2004

15. "Minnesota Business Partnerships testifies in support of State Imposed Health Care Rationing" Citizens' Council on Health Care, May 15, 2003. www.cchc-mn.org/pr/pr051303.php

16. "Minnesota Rx Connect: Minnesota's Plan". www.state.mn.us/cgi-bin/portal/mn/jsp/content.do?id=536885154&agency=rx2004

17. "Mn Best Practices Law" Chapter 288 Governor Pawlenty May 29, 2004". [Citizens' Council on Health Care]. www.cchconline.org June 2004.

18. www.maximumstrengthhealthcare.com/qa.html 2004

19. "Medicine Cabinet/Exerting State Leadership". Star Tribune Editorial, May 30, 2004 www.maximumstrengthhealthcare.com/editorial5-29-2004.html

20. "Health Care Costs: Governor's Health Cabinet flexing state muscle". Pioneer Plus Editorial. May 16, 2004. www.maximumstrengthhealthcare.com/editorial5-16-2004.html 2004

21. www.dhs.state.mn.us/main/groups/healthcare/documents/pub/dhs_id_006926.hcsp

22. www.dhs.state.mn.us/main/groups/healthcare/documents/pub/dhs_id_006927.hcsp

23. www.dhs.state.mn.us/main/groups/healthcare/documents/pub/dhs_id_006932.hcsp

24. www.dhs.state.mn.us/main/groups/healthcare/documents/pub/dhs_id_006933.hcsp

25. www.dhs.state.mn.us/main/groups/healthcare/documents/pub/
    dhs_id_006924.hcsp

26. www.dhs.state.mn.us/main/groups/healthcare/documents/pub/
    dhs_id_006925.hcsp

27. www.dhs.state.mn.us/main/groups/healthcare/documents/pub/
    dhs_id_006930.hcsp

28. www.dhs.state.mn.us/main/groups/healthcare/documents/pub/
    dhs_id_006928.hcsp

29. www.dhs.state.mn.us/main/groups/healthcare/documents/pub/
    dhs_id_006271.hcsp

30. www.dhs.state.mn.us/main/groups/healthcare/documents/pub/
    dhs_id_006254.hcsp

31. www.dhs.state.mn.us/main/groups/healthcare/documents/pub/
    dhs_id_006258.hcsp

32. www.mass.gov/healthcare

33. "HHS Approves Plan to Save Money on Prescription Drugs". United States Department of Health and Human Services, September 9, 2004. www.hhs.gov/news/press/2004pres/20040909a.html

34. "Doctor Visits replaced by Paramedics" BBC Look North East Yorkshire/ Lincolnshire January 14,2005

35. "More Uninsured as Oregon Health Plan Withers" Sullivan, Niki: Associated Press, January 18, 2005. KATU.com Oregon 2005

36. "Oregon Health Plan Faces New Cuts on Thursday" Associated Press, June 27, 2004. KATU.com Oregon 2004

37. "Oregon Health Plan in Critical Condition" Gustafson, Alan. Statesman Journal.com 2003. http://newsstatesmanjournal.com/article.cfm?i=69072

38. "Doctors Refuse to See Oregon Health Plan Patients". Kramer, Andrew. Associated Press, September 23, 2003. KATU.com Oregon 2003. www.katu.com/news/story.asp?ID=60916

39. "Proposed Beer Tax Would Fund Alcohol Addiction Programs", Cain, Brad: Associated Press, Feb.11, 2005. KATU.com Oregon 2005. www.katu.com/news/story.asp?ID=74860

40. "New Certified Plans Information" State of Oregon Insurance Pool Governing Board. 2005. www.ipgb.state.or.us 2005

41. "First Pass Initiative for Medicaid Claims Processing". http://oregon.gov/DHS/healthplan/first-pass/main.shtml/ Oregon DHS Website 2004

42. "Governor Introduces New Health Insurance Plan". Dornfield, Ann. Associated Press 2005. KMTR Oregon 2005. www.kmtr.com/news/local/story.aspx?content_id=FOA2859E-9242-4F11-B639-BF430FOE27ABD

43. "Smith Wants Creation of Medicaid Panel". Associated Press 2005. KMTR Oregon 2005. www.kmtr.com/news/local/story.aspx?content_id=85870A24-8CC7-4536-A075-900201A838BC

44. "Medical Marijuana Cards Booming": Associated Press 2005. KMTR Oregon 2005. www.kmtr.com/news/local/story.aspx?content_id=8341C6CC-22DE-4A69-BC/1-C1218FF84FC5

45. "Group Seeks to Stop Health Plan Funding of Abortion". Associated Press 2005. Oregonian 2005. KMTR Oregon 2005. www.kmtr.com/news/state/story.aspx?content_id=AF19A820-25D4-4845-B223-2041028ED994

46. "Legislators: Health Care Systems Could Get Incremental Fixes". Associated Press 2005. KMTR Oregon 2005. www.kmtr.com/news/state/story.aspx?content_id=A6B441FF-2EEB-41BC-B856A74418B05223

47. "Governor Pawlenty and the Mayo Clinic Decline to Participate: Only Public Forum on Governor's Genetic Research Initiative is cancelled". Media Release Citizens' Council on Health Care February 14, 2005. www.cchconline.org/pr/021405.php

48. "Home Care Advisory Work Group: Recommendations to Change Regulations that Will Maintain and Improve the Quality and Delivery of Home

Care Services to Minnesotans. Report to Minnesota Legislature". State of Minnesota Department of Health 2005. http://www.health.state.mn.us/divs/fpc/HClegrpt05.pdf

49. "The Truth about Tenncare" Tennesseans for Fair Taxation. 2002-2004. http://www.yourtax.org/facts/tenncare.php3

50. http://www.ichope.com/index.cgi?token=10352010181&page=mplate.tenncare.html Mental Health Association of Middle Tennessee 2002.

51. "Applying for Tenncare". State of Tennessee Bureau of Tenncare 2005. http://www.tennessee.gov/tenncare/howdoI.html

52. "Doctors, Hospitals can check Tenncare Elligibility Online at Tennesee.org". Stae of Tennessee Bureau of Tenncare: Nashville, Tennessee 2001. http://www.tennessee.gov/tenncare/elligibilityverificationonline.html

53. "Tenncare Pharmacy". State of Tennessee Bureau of Tenncare 2005. http://www.tennessee.gov/tenncare/pharminfo.html

54. "Turkmen Leader Closes Hospital". Whitlock, Monica. BBC News 2005. http://news.bbc.co.uk/1/hi/world/asia-pacific/4307583

55. Ministries: Ministry of Public Health and Medical Industry of Turkmenistan 2005. http://www.tacistm.org/Ministries/Ministries%20al/htm

56. "Report: Number of Minnesotans without Health Insurance Jumps". Associated Press February 26, 2005. wcco.com.

57. "Six Insurance Plans to be offered for Uninsured". Associated Press January 27, 2005. wcco.com. http://wcco.com/localnews/local_story_027200229.html

58. "Proposed Bill seeks to limit Hospital Bills for Uninsured". Associated Press February 9, 2005. wcco.com. http://wcco.com/localnews/local_story_040184412.html

59. "Legislature 05: Rising Health Costs Pressure some Benefits". Associated Press January 1, 2005. wcco.com. http://wcco.com/localnews/local_story_001160050.html

60. "Pawlenty Health Cuts would raise uncompensated Hospital Care". Associated Press January 26, 2005. WCCO.com http://wcco.com/localnews/local_story_026183127.html

61. "Hospital Charity Care Practices Challenged". Associated Press November 27, 2004. WCCO.com. http://wcco.com/localnews/local_story_332162653.html

62. "I Team: Comparing Hospital Care Costs". WCCO March 2, 2005. http://wcco.com/localnews/local_story_061192832.html

63. "Pawlenty Floats Idea of Using Tribes to Import Drugs". Associated Press February 16, 2005. WCCO.com. http://wcco.com/localnews/local_story_047144638.html/resources_storyPrintableView

64. "MN Drug Program with Canada Expanding". Associated Press February 4, 2005. WCCO.com. http://wcco.com/localnews/local_story_035071642.html/resources_storyPrintableView

65. "Seniors Look beyond Canada for Drugs". Associated Press February 28, 2005. WCCO.com http://wcco.com/localnews/local_story_058181311.html/resources_storyPrintableView

66. "Pawlenty Considers Drug Imports from Britain" Associated Press March 10, 2005. WCCO.com. http://wcco.com/localnews/local_story_069111312.html/resources_storyPrintableView

67. "Pawlenty to Announce Prescription Plan Including Europe". Associated Press March 15, 2005. WCCO.com. http://wcco.com/localnews/local_story_074143827.html/resources_storyPrintableView

68. "Changing Tenncare in an Adversarial Legal Environment" Tenncare 2004

69. "Organ Panel Approves Mental Health Parity Measure". Beggs, Charles E. Associated Press March 10, 2005. http://www.kgw.com/health/stories/kgw_031005_health_mental_health.1248d008d.html

70. "House Bill 955: Comprehensive Study on Health Care and Health Care Costs in New Mexico". State of New Mexico Legislative Health and Human Services Committee: Santa Fe, New Mexico December 2004. legis.state.nm.us/lcs/lcsdocs/153454.pdf

71. "Few Americans Use Internet to buy Prescription Drugs". Associated Press October 11, 2004. WCCO.com. http://wcco.com/localnews/local_story_285974931.html/resources_storyPrintableView

72. "Bill would require Health Insurance in 2007" Associated Press March 29, 2005/WCCO.com http://wcco.com/localnews/local_story_088142746.html/resources_storyPrintableView

73. "Senate Votes to Sign Health Care Caps". Associated Press March 31, 2005. WCCO. Com http://wcco.com/localnews/local_story_090131801.html/resources_storyPrintableView

74. "Senate Votes to Restore some Health Care Funding". Associated Press April 1, 2005. WCCO.com http://wcco.com/localnews/local_story_091094049.html/resources_storyPrintableView

75. "Drug Boards Voting on Import Issue". Associated Press April 4, 2005. WCCO.com http://wcco.com/localnews/local_story_094160031.html/resources_storyPrintableView

76. "AARP Drug Costs Jump in 2004". Associated Press April 12, 2005. WCCO.com http://wcco.com/localnews/local_story_102111550.html/resources_storyPrintableView

77. "Minnesota Leads Nation in Health Insurance Coverage". Associated Press April 27, 2005. WCCO.com http://wcco.com/localnews/local_story_116213429.html

78. "IBM Plans to start Network for Health Care Data". Associated Press April 24, 2005. WCCO.com http://wcco.com/localnews/local_story_114191032.html

79. "Shareholders Reject MN Drug Import Resolution". Associated Press May 4, 2005. WCCO.com http://wcco.com/localnews/local_story_124132336.html

80. "Senate Approves Health Bill with Minnesota Care Expansion". Associated Press May 4, 2005. WCCO.com http://wcco.com/localnews/local_story_12416236.html

81. "Fire Crew Replacing Paramedics". BBC News 2002. http://news.bbc.co.uk/1/hi/health/2163185.stm

82. "Ambulance Cover Hit by Sickness". BBC News 2005. http://news.bbc.co.uk/1/hi/england/southern_counties/3490930.stm

83. "Ambulance Service in Meltdown". BBC News 2005. http://news.bbc.co.uk/1/hi/england/kent4339481.stm

84. "NHS Waiting Lists Up in January". BBC News 2005. http://news.bbc.co.uk/1/hi/health/4339959.stm

85. "MRSA did not cause Hospital Death"/BBC News April 14, 2005. http://news.bbc.co.uk/go/pr/fr/-/1/hi/england/devon/4445197.stm

86. "Hospital Acres Sold For Housing". BBC News May 24, 2005. http://news.bbc.co.uk/1/hi/england/norfolk/4574691.stm

87. Report on Hospital Targets by BBC Spotlight [was seen on Real Player by the Underwriter] on April 14, 2005. http://www.bbc.co.uk/devon/mediaplayer/spotlight.shtml

88. "NHS and Pacemakers" BBC Midlands Today [Seen on Real Player by the Underwriter on May 27, 2005]

89. Comments on NHS: Interview with Community Health Council on the Alan Beswick Show. [Heard by the Underwriter on Real Player May 13, 2005].

90. "GOP Candidate Unveils Health Proposals" Boston.com. 2006. http://www.boston.com/news/local/maine/articles/2006/03/24/gop_candidate_unveils_health_care_proposals

91. "Wisconsin Badger Care, Badger Care at a Glance" State of Wisconsin Department of Health and Family Services; February 2005. Assessed on March 28, 2005

92. http://www.dhfs.state.wi.us/badgercare/html/glance-2.htm

93. http://www.dhfs.state.wi.us/badgercare/html/gl ance-3.htm

94. http://www.dhfs.state.wi.us/badgercare/html/gl ance-4.htm

95. "Report: One in Four Nursing Homes at Risk of Closing" http://wcco.com/
health/local story 085105924.html/resources storyPrintableView

96. "Britain gets MN Nod for Cheaper Prescriptions". Associated Press 2005.
WCCO.com.   http://wcco.com/siteSearch/local story 077093238.html/
resources storyPrintableView

97. "The Potential Impact of Eliminating Tenncare and reverting to Medicaid:
A Preliminary Analysis". Kay, L; Wachino, V. Center on Budeget and Policy
Priorities. November 15, 2004. http://www.cbpp.org/11-15-04health.htm

98. "Religious Group Joins Tenncare Sit In". WSMV.com June 23, 2005.
http://www.wsmv.com/Global/story.asp?S=3514238&nav=1TcRbOIW

99. "Tenncare Protestors plan Third Ovenight Vigil at Governor's Office".
Associated Press June 22, 2005.WSMV.com. http://www.wsmv.
com/Global/story.asp?S=3507624

100."Nurses Protest against Health Care Ruling". CBC News June 10, 2005.
cbc.ca.   http://montreal/cbc.ca/regional/servlet/View?filename=qc-
nurses20050610

101."Some Experts Expect Tenncare change to affect other patients". Associated
Press February 11, 2005. WSMV.com. http://www.wsmv.com/Global/
story.asp?S=2935196&ClientType=Printable

102."Tenncare Changes could mean rate hike at Hospitals". Associated Press
February 13, 2005. wsmv.com. http://www.wsmv.com/Global/
story.asp?S=2940270

103."Poll: Governor's Approval Rating High, but Tenncare opinions mixed".
Associated Press February 17, 2005. wsmv.com. http://www.wsmv.com/
Global/story.asp?S=2966157&ClientType=Printable

104."Tenncare Lawyers ask Appeals Court to rule without a hearing". Associated
Press February 18, 2005. wsmv.com. http://www.wsmv.com/Global/
story.asp?S=2969530&ClientType=Printable

105. "Senator balks when Tenncare syas he must pay $75,000 for Records". Associated Press February 23, 2005.wsmv.com. http://www.wsmv.com/Global/story.asp?S=2989411&ClientType=Printable

106. "Senator Ford files complaints against TV Station Reporter". Associated Press February 25, 2005. wmsv.com. http://www.wsmv.com/Global/story.asp?S=2994906&ClientType=Printable

107. "State Investigates Ford's ties to Tenncare Money". Associated Press February 24, 2005. wsmv.com. http://www.wsmv.com/Global/story.asp?S=2996073&ClientType=Printable

108. "Fords have been investigated before over ties to Tenncare Money". Associated Press March 17, 2005. wsmv.com. http://www.wsmv.com/Global/story.asp?S=3000834&ClientType=Printable

109. "Attorney General asked to investigate Ford-Ternncare Ties". Associated Press March 3, 2005.wsmv.com. Dagny, Stewart. http://www.wsmv.com/Global/story.asp?S=3010342&ClientType=Printable

110. "Activist asks FBI to look into Tenncare Allegations". Associated Press March 7, 2005. wsmv.com. Cole, Karen. http://www.wsmv.com/Global/story.asp?S=3011458&ClientType=Printable

111. "Tenncare Enrollee's Lawyer tells Court problem is management". Associated Press March 28, 2005. wsmv.com. http://www.wsmv.com/Global/story.asp?S=3131185&ClientType=Printable

112. "Republican Leaders focus on Bredesen's Handling of Tenncare". Associated Press March 31, 2005.wsmv.com. http://www.wsmv.com/Global/story.asp?S=3152076&ClientType=Printable

113. "Health Officials say Tenncare Cuts could hurt Hospitals". Associated Press March 31, 2005. wsmv.com. http://www.wsmv.com/Global/story.asp?S=3141083&ClientType=Printable

114. "Spinning Wheels". Blood, Sweat, and Tears from the CD "What Goes Up: The Best of Blood, Sweat, and Tears". Sony Records Catalog #64166. ASIN B000002A2Y

115. "Number of Uninsured Children reaches a five year high in Tennessee". Associated Press February 7, 2005. wsmv.com. http://www.wsmv. com/Global/story.asp?S=29

116. "Judges Rejects Ban of Justice Center In Tenncare Case". Associated Press February 10, 2005. wsmv.comhttp://www.wsmv.com/Global/ story.asp?S=2929704&ClientType=Printable

117. "AARP proposes Alternative Reform to Tenncare". Associated Press February 10, 2005. wsmv.com. http://www.wsmv.com/Global/ story.asp?S=2931167&ClientType=Printable

118. "Former Tenncare Director says cutting rolls, fighting fraud needed". Associated Press April 5, 2005. wsmv.com. http://www.wsmv.com/Global/ story.asp?S=3170772&ClientType=Printable

119. "Tenncare hearing postponed two days". Associated Press April 4, 2005. wsmv.com. http://www.wsmv.com/Global/story. asp?S=3164350&ClientType=Printable

120. "Bredesen: "Safety Net will protect those cut from Tenncare" Associated Press April 20, 2005. wsmv.com. http://www.wsmv.com/Global/ story.asp?S=3238606&ClientType=Printable

121. "Tenncare looking to replace contractor with ties to Ford." Associated Press April 20, 2005. wsmv.com. http://www.wsmv.com/Global/ story.asp?S=3236794&ClientType=Printable

122. "Judge delays Tenncare Case to await word from Federal Officials". Associated Press April 20, 2005. wsmv.com. http://www.wsmv.com/Global/ story.asp?S=32381938&ClientType=Printable

123. "Bush to push Sweeping Health Reform". Perry, Candace Phyiscans News Digest January 2003. http://www.physiciansnews.com/cover/103.html

124. "Senator Ford tells paper he won't seek reelection". Associated Press May 7, 2005. wsmv.com. http://www.wsmv.com/Global/story. asp?S=3314438&ClientType=Printable

125. "Federal Government files brief in favor of Tenn Cuts". Associated Press 2005. wsmv.com. http://www.wsmv.com/Global/story.asp?S=3358466

126. "Governor Takes Issue with Contingency Plan" Associated Press 2005. wsmv.com.
http://www.wsmv.com/Global/story.asp?S=33775098&nav=1TcRa9x1

127. "Lawmakers concerned New Tenncare Investigator has no conviction" Associated Press 2005. wsmv.com. http://www.wsmv.com/Global/story.asp?S=3377489

128. "Officials en enrollment for some Tenncare Programs". Associated Press 2005. wsmv.com. http://www.wsmv.com/Global/story/.asp?S=3274982

129. "State ready to send disenrollment notices". Associated Press 2005. wsmv.com. http://wsmv.com/global/story.asp?s=3407316&ClientType=Printable

130. "Public Hospitals to be hit hardest when Tenncare Cuts Rolls". Associated Press 2005. wsmv.com. http://wsmv.com/global/story.asp?s=3409003&ClientType=Printable

131. "Facing Bribery Charges, John Ford resigns from Senate Seat". Associated Press 2005. wsmv.com http://wsmv.com/global/story.asp?s=3404654

132. "Judge sets Tenncare hearing for end of month". Associated Press 2005. wsmv.com. http://www.wsmv.com/global/story.asp?s=3437571&ClientType=Printable

133. "Lawmakers: Voters should force Legislature to act on Health Care". Associated Press 2005. Clear Channel Communications 2005. nbc16.com. http://www.nbc16.com/common/printstory/default.aspx?content_id=c9d5cbe4-77bf-451f-a

134. "Nevadans may soon have a choice to buy Canadian Drugs Online". Patterson, Lindsey May 13, 2005@0130AM KLAS-TV.com. http://www.klas-tv.com/Global/story.asp?S=3332919&nav=168XWZRT

135. "Bills sail through Nevada Legislature Deadline". Associated Press 2005. KLAS-TV.com. http://www.klas-tv.com/Global/story.asp?S=3265150

136. "Hospital Bills for Illegal Immigrants: Who Pays?" Mc Carty, Colleen, May 12, 2005. KLAS-TV.com http://www.klas-tv.com/Global/story.asp?S=3332745&nav=168YzkrD

137. "An Option for Cheaper Prescription Drugs". Platt, Sarah. World Now 2005. wkbt.com. http://www.wkbt.com/global/story.asp?s=3151711&ClientType=Printable

138. "Washington Senate passes major mental health reform bill". Associated Press March 11, 2005. kgw.com. http://www.kgw.com/health/stories/kgw_031105_health_mental_health.12ada5da.html

139. "GOP Lawmakers toast Health Insurance Initiatives". Associated Press 2005. WLBZ 2 March 15, 2005. http://www.wlbz2.com/search/article.asp?id=20947

140. "High Tech Video Conference to be held on Health Care". Associated Press 2005. WLBZ 2 March 11, 2005. http://www.wlbz2.com/search/article.asp?id=20858

141. "Introduction to the Review of Legislation" Florida State University Law Review 1996. http://www.law.fsu.edu/journals/lawreview/issues/232/chiles.html

142. "Governor Bush: Reforms for Quality Health Care". Miami Herald April 7, 2003. MyFlorida.com. http://www.myflorida.com/myflorida/government/mediacenter/edletters/03/reform-0407-03.html

143. "Ruling Halts Cuts of Tenncare Rolls". Wadhwani, Anita, January 29, 2005. The Tennessean.com. http://www.tennessean.com/government/tenncare/archives/05/01/64802477.shtml?element

144. "Bredesen slices benefits to 719,000 on Tenncare". Wadhwani, Anita, January 29, 2005. The Tennessean.com. http://www.tennessean.com/government/tenncare/archives/05/01/63956952.shtml?element

145. "Maine". The World Book Encyclopedia: M Volume 13, page 70. World Book Inc. A Scott Fetzer Company. Chicago, Illinois 2000

146. "FAQ's & Glossary of Dirigo Health Terms". Dirigo Health 2003. Pages 1-6. http://dirigohealth.maine.gov/dhsp01d.html

147. "Providing Health Insurance is good for Business". Dirigo Health 2003. Pages 1-3. http://dirigohealth.maine.gov/dhsp02a.html

148. "Maine Quality Forum: Your Guide to High Quality Health Care". Dirigo Health 2003. Pages 1-3. http://dirigohealth.maine.gov/dhsp06.html

149. "Leading the Way?" News Hour with Jim Lehrer Transcript November 26, 2003. pgs.1-7. http://www.pbs.org/newshour/bb/health/july-dec03/maine_12-1.html

150. "Crossing the Quality Chasm: A New Health System for the 21st Century". Institute of Medicine 2001. http://www.iom.edu/report.asp?id=5432

151. "Mi Rx Prescription Savings Program". www.michigan.gov/som/0,1607,7-192-29942_32789-100833—,00.html

152. "States take up their own Health Care Reform". Lamb, Gregory M. June 10, 2004. The Christian Science Monitor. http://www.csmonitor.com/2004/0610/p11s01-uspo.html

153. "Arizona State Wide Health Reform Demonstration" Center for Medicare & Medicaid Services. 2004. http://www.cms.hhs.gov/medicaid/1115/azfact.asp

154. "Real Health Care Reform". Johnson, Senator Steve. June 11, 2003. ColoradoSenate.com. http://www.coloradosenate.com/results.php3?news_id=382

155. "Governor Baldacci Announces Hospital Commission" State of Maine Office of Health Policy and Finance 2003. http://www.maine.gov/governor/baldacci/healthpolicy/news/10_9_03.htm

156. "Governor Names Dirigo Health Board of Directors" State of Maine Office of Health Policy and Finance 2003. http://www.maine.gov/governor/baldacci/healthpolicy/news/9_5_03.htm

157. "Governor Baldacci unveils plans for Minnesota Rx Plus" State of Maine Office of Health Policy and Finance 2003. http://www.maine.gov/governor/baldacci/healthpolicy/news/5_30_03.htm

158. "Governor Baldacci signs Executive Order creating Office of Health Policy and Finance" State of Maine Office of Health Policy and Finance 2003. http://www.maine.gov/governor/baldacci/healthpolicy/news/1_9_03.htm

159. "Governor Baldacci and Office of Health Policy and Finance announce Prescription Drug Plan for Great Northern Workers" State of Maine Office of Health Policy and Finance 2003. http://www.maine.gov/governor/baldacci/healthpolicy/news/3_5_03.htm

160. "Governor Announces Task Force on Veterans Health Care" State of Maine Office of Health Policy and Finance 2003. http://www.maine.gov/governor/baldacci/healthpolicy/news/11_7_03.htm

161. "Dirigo Health Reform Shows Early Success" State of Maine Office of Health Policy and Finance 2003. http://www.maine.gov/governor/baldacci/healthpolicy/news/12_22_03.htm

162. "Dirigo Health Appoints Executive Director" Office of Health Policy and Finance 2004. http://www.maine.gov/governor/baldacci/healthpolicy/news/1_9_04.htm

163. "Brief History of Reform" Office of Health Policy and Finance 2005. http://www.me.gov/governor/baldacci/healthpolicy/news/what_is_dirigo_health/index.html2005

164. "Governor Announces Brochure to help Mainers Compare Hospital Prices" Office of Health Policy and Finance 2004. http://www.maine.gov/governor/baldacci/healthpolicy/news/1_27_04.htm

165. "Governor Announces New Dirigo Health Brochure" Office of Health Policy and Finance 2004. http://www.maine.gov/governor/baldacci/healthpolicy/news/2_13_04.htm

166. "Governor announces selection of Maine Physician to direct Maine Quality Forum" Office of Health Policy and Finance 2004. http://www.maine.gov/governor/baldacci/healthpolicy/news/3_12_04.htm

167. "Governor Announces Initiative to Assist Medicare Beneficiaries access prescription cards" Office of Health Policy and Finance 2004. http://www.maine.gov/governor/baldacci/healthpolicy/news/4_28_04.htm

168. "Dirigo Health Agency releases RFP, seeks carriers to offer Dirigo Health Plan" Office of Health Policy and Finance 2004. http://www.maine.gov/governor/baldacci/healthpolicy/news/5_7_04.htm

169. "Dirigo Choice helping more working families" Office of Health Policy and Finance 2005. http://www.maine.gov/governor/baldacci/healthpolicy/news/5_2_05.htm

170. "Dirigo Health Reform receives major support from local health foundation" Office of Health Policy and Finance 2004. http://www.maine.gov/governor/baldacci/healthpolicy/news/5_13_04.htm

171. "Dirigo Health Plan receives bid from Anthem" Office of Health Policy and Finance 2004. http://www.maine.gov/governor/baldacci/healthpolicy/news/6_11_04.htm

172. "Dirigo Health has successful first year" Office of Health Policy and Finance 2004.   http://www.me.gov/governor/baldacci/healthpolicy/news/9_13_04.htm

173. "Maine Quality Forum Website goes online" Office of Health Policy and Finance 2004. http://www.me.gov/governor/baldacci/healthpolicy/news/11_15_04.htm

174. "Hospital releases Draft Report for Public Comment" Office of Health Policy and Finance 2004. http://www.me.gov/governor/baldacci/healthpolicy/news/12_22_04.htm

175. "State Health Plan Released" Office of Health Policy and Finance 2004. http://www.me.gov/governor/baldacci/healthpolicy/news/7_26_04.htm

176. "Governor's Office Issues Emergency Rules to establish Capital Investment Funds after significant public input" Office of Health Policy and Finance 2004.   http://www.me.gov/governor/baldacci/healthpolicy/news/7_27_04.htm

177. "Capital Investment Fund Amount Released" Office of Health Policy and Finance 2004. http://www.me.gov/governor/baldacci/healthpolicy/news/8_6_04.htm

178. "Ad Campaign to raise awareness of Dirigo Health Reform" Office of Health Policy and Finance 2004. http://www.me.gov/governor/baldacci/healthpolicy/news/8_16_04.htm

179. "Governor announces Dirigo Choice Agreement" Office of Health Policy and Finance 2004. http://www.me.gov/governor/baldacci/healthpolicy/news/8_23_04.htm

180. "Health Care Reform Efforts Win Praise" Greenberg, Scott S; April 7, 2005. The Boston Globe

181. "Wisonsin Legislative Update May 2004" Wisconsin Women's Network. http://www.wiwomensnetwork.org/stateleg.html#signed

182. "Public Health Restructuring Report". Nelson, Helene; February 3, 2004. State of Wisconsin Department of Health and Family Services. http://www.dhfs.wisconsin.gov

183. "Consumer Directed Health Care". Healthology Inc. 2005. http://www.wfrv.healthology.com http://www.wfrv.healthology.com/printer_friendly.asp?f=healthcare&c=healthcare_patientdirect

184. "2005-2007 DHFS Items included in the Governor's Biennial Budget February 8, 2005, revised February 23, 2005" State of Wisconsin 2005, pages 1-10.

185. "SB9" Nevada State Legislature 2005. http://leg.state.nv.us/73rd/Report/histort.cf?ID=1299

186. "Santa Fe Indian Hospital Have Health Care Shortages" Associated Press May 24, 2005. KOB TV.com. http://www.kobtv.com/index.cfm?viewer=storyviewer&id=19373&cat=4HEALTH

187. "Albuquerque Hospital Phasing Out Adult Hospice Program" Associated Press April 30, 2005. KOB TV.com. http://www.kobtv.com/index.cfm?viewer=storyviewer&id=18834&cat=4HEALTH

188. "Advocates say UNM Hospital denying care to poor." Associated Press May 7, 2005. KOB TV.com. http://www.kobtv.com/index.cfm?viewer=storyviewer&id=18989&cat=4HEALTH

189. "2003 House Bill for HB 0489" New Mexico State Legislature 2003. http://legis.state.nm.us/sessions/03%20regular/bills/house/HB0498

190. "Medical Insecurity: Why We Need the New Mexico Health Care Plan" Blume, June 2001. Health Security for New Mexico Campaign. http://www.nmhealthsecurity.org/back/nm_back.html

191. "Summary of the 2003 New Mexico Health Security Act" http://www.nmhealthsecurity.org/back/nm_theplan.html

192. "Why the New Mexico Health Security Plan is Necessary" http://www.nmhealthsecurity.org/plan.nm_fs1.htm

193. "The New Mexico Health Security Act" http://www.nmhealthsecurity.org/plan.nm_fs2.htm

194. "The New Mexico Health Security Plan: A Plan that makes good business sense". http://www.nmhealthsecurity.org/plan.nm_fs3.htm

195. "The Canadian Cure" Kraker, Daniel. 2001 The New Rules Project. http://www.newrules.org/journal/nrwin01health.html

196. "Canadian Health Care System" www.newrules.org http://www.newrules.org/equity/CNhealthcare.html

197. "Canada Health Act" Department of Jsutice Canada. http://laws.justice.gc.ca/en/c-6/17077.html

198. "The Court Strikes Down Quebec Private Health Care Law" CBC News June 9, 2005. cbc.ca http://ottawa.cbc.ca/regional/servlet/View?filename=ot-sco2005609

199. "Gatineau Doctor Welcomes Health Ruling" CBC News June 9, 2005. cbc.ca http://ottawa.cbc.ca/regional/servlet/View?filename=ot-gathealth2005609

200. "Group Worried by Health Care Decisions" CBC News June 10, 2005. cbc.ca http://ottawa.cbc.ca/regional/servlet/View?filename=pe_health_20056010

201. "Judge sets Tenncare hearing for end of month". Associated Press 2005. wsmv.com. http://www.wsmv.com/global/story. asp?s=3437571&ClientType=Printable

202. "Ruling Halts Cuts of Tenncare Rolls". Wadhwani, Anita, January 29, 2005. The Tennessean.com. http://www.tennessean.com/government/ tenncare/archives/05/01/64802477.shtml?element

203. "Bredesen slices benefits to 719,000 on Tenncare". Wadhwani, Anita, January 29, 2005. The Tennessean.com. http://www.tennessean. com/government/tenncare/archives/05/01/63956952.shtml?element

204. "Governor Fletcher Outlines Medicaid Changes". WAVE 3; Associated Press. 2006. http://www.wave3.com/Global/story.asp?s=4379816

205. "Ky Health Choices" Kentucky: Cabinet for Health and Family Services. 2006.

206. "Appeals Court says Medicaid Patients can sue" Associated Press. KGW 2006. http://www.kgw.com/cgi-bin/bi/gold_print.cgi

207. "Kulongoski Pushes Affordable Health Care Focus" Associated Press. KGW 2006.
http://www.kgw.com/election2002/stories/
kgw_020906_health_kulongski_care.dce5719...

208. "Kulongoski unveils health,school,environment plans" Associated Press. KGW 2006.
http://www.kgw.com/eductaion/localeducation/stories/
kgw_020406_news_state_of_state.5

209. "Ashland Doctor to Lead Oregon Health Plan". Associated Press. KGW 2006. http://www.kgw.com/cgi-bin/bi/gold_print.cgi

210. "Governor's Fit City Program" Minnesota Department of Health. 2006. http://www.health.state.mn.us/fitcity

211. "Rose Garden". Lynn Anderson. Brentwood Records. [Audio CD 2005]. B0008FPJBW

212. "Rose Garden". Joe South. Raven Records. [Audio CD 2005]. B00000JG1Q

213. "A Good Start: The House Health Care Reform Bills" Haislmaier, Edmund F; Moffit, Robert E. Ph.D; Owcharenko,Nina. Web Memo: The Heritage Foundation. Web Memo #803 July 22, 2005 http://www.heritage.org/Research/HealthCare/wm803.cfm?renderforprint=1

ABOUT THE AUTHOR

Dr. Alvarez-Galloso graduated from Universidad Central Del Este [in the Dominican Republic] with a Degree of Doctor in Medicine. After his graduation, Dr. Alvarez-Galloso decided to pursue his studies in the Administrative Realm of Medicine. Mr. Alvarez-Galloso passed the Certification Examination for Utilization Review [which is administered by Mc Kesson Inter Qual*]. Dr. Alvarez-Galloso has given lectures on Medical Documentation to diverse members of Multidisciplinary Teams in Hospital Settings. In the year 2004, his first book "Defensive Documentation and More/Documentation Preventive" was published by Page Free Publishing/RKD Press.

978-0-595-39445-6
0-595-39445-0

www.ingramcontent.com/pod-product-compliance
Lightning Source LLC
Chambersburg PA
CBHW051447280526
45785CB00003B/1469